WE ALL LIVE IN THE HOT ZONE NOW

Antibiotics have failed. With the coming of exotic new viruses, and the evolution of microbes resistant to the drugs we've used for the last fifty years, we have never needed an alternative therapy more.

Olive leaf extract—effective, natural, and nontoxic—has been used as a folk remedy for thousands of years. Only now has scientific research shown that the active ingredient, *oleuropein,* has vast healing powers because it actually eliminates the viruses, fungi, bacteria, and other parasites that cause disease.

From immune disorders to the common cold, from athlete's foot to malaria, olive leaf extract can be a powerful adjunct to any program of healing, health, and wellness.

BOOK YOUR PLACE ON OUR WEBSITE AND MAKE THE READING CONNECTION!

We've created a customized website just for our very special readers, where you can get the inside scoop on everything that's going on with Zebra, Pinnacle and Kensington books.

When you come online, you'll have the exciting opportunity to:

- View covers of upcoming books

- Read sample chapters

- Learn about our future publishing schedule (listed by publication month *and author*)

- Find out when your favorite authors will be visiting a city near you

- Search for and order backlist books from our online catalog

- Check out author bios and background information

- Send e-mail to your favorite authors

- Meet the Kensington staff online

- Join us in weekly chats with authors, readers and other guests

- Get writing guidelines

- AND MUCH MORE!

Visit our website at
http://www.kensingtonbooks.com

OLIVE LEAF EXTRACT

DR. MORTON WALKER

Foreword by
Joseph J. Territo, M.D.

Kensington Books
Kensington Publishing Corp.
http://www.kensingtonbooks.com

KENSINGTON BOOKS are published by

Kensington Publishing Corp.
850 Third Avenue
New York, NY 10022

Kensington and the K logo Reg. U.S. Pat. & TM Off.

First Kensington Paperback Printing: November, 1997
10 9 8 7 6

Printed in the United States of America

To Kensington Publishing acquisition and development editor **Lee Heiman,** who ferrets out health-related subjects of vital interest, finds the authors to address them, and guides the projects into informative books for the medical consumer. That's what Lee did for this book.

Acknowledgments

Recognition should be given to William R. Fredrickson for his pioneering research and development of olive leaf extract as a treatment for infectious diseases. The current interest in the use of olive leaf extract has been primarily stimulated by the ongoing work of Mr. Fredrickson throughout the last decade.

Disclaimer

This book has been written and published strictly for informational purposes. In no way should it be used as a substitute for your own physician's advice. The author, Morton Walker, D.P.M., is not practicing as a health professional but rather is reporting on health care information that he has researched as a medical journalist.

You should not consider educational material in this book to be the practice of medicine, although almost all the facts have come from research of the world's published medical literature on olive trees, olives, olive oil, olive leaves, olive bark, and other olive tree-related products; plus the files and personal interviews of informed health professionals diagnosing and treating illnesses and/or their patients who have suffered from such illnesses.

Except for those people mentioned in Chapter 8, whose stories are taken from *Positive Health News* and the book *How to Reverse Immune Dysfunction,* written by Mark Konlee and published by Keep Hope Alive, the identities of patients volunteering personal health-related stories are hidden. Although every individual providing an experience with olive leaf extract gave permission for his or her name and location to be used, it's this author's preference to protect the identities of these people. Apart from the HIV-positive persons who want their stories told, the names of patients are pseudonyms as are their locations and occupations. Still, facts and personal histories about all patients' illnesses are stated as they were revealed during the author's tape-recorded interviews with them.

If you, as a potential user of the information in this book, require opinions, diagnoses, treatments, therapeutic advice, correction of your lifestyle, or any other aid relating to your health, it is recommended by the author and the publisher that you consult your own medical expert.

These statements are to be considered disclaimers of responsibility for anything published here. The author and publisher provide the information in this book with the understanding that you may act on it at your own risk and also with full knowledge that health professionals should first be consulted and that their specific advice for you should be considered before anything read here.

This book reflects the views of Dr. Morton Walker. While others may disagree with these views, they are based on sound and reliable reports. Nothing in this book should be considered a claim for any specific product.

Contents

PART ONE

The Developmental History of the Therapeutic Attributes of Olive Leaf Extract

PART TWO

Successful Antimicrobial Therapy for Viral, Bacterial, Fungal, and Parasitic Illnesses

Foreword

Historically, an olive branch has symbolized compromise and peace between opposing parties.

Fruit from this tree, the olive, and its juice, olive oil, have assumed stellar roles in the culinary world. They are nourishing and delicious foods, and offer many health benefits.

Today, we are learning to appreciate the importance of still another part of the olive tree—the olive leaf—and its role as a medicinal product, which is bringing betterment to all humankind.

From the earliest days of recorded history, reference has been made to properties of the olive tree. Look at olive oil, for instance. While it's true that olive oil was used in the kitchen because it enhanced food, we now know that its medicinal properties played a part as well. Without doubt, consuming olive oil improves health and longevity.

In today's society, the physician's role has altered dramatically from what it had been only fifty years ago. Medical doctors, and some other health professionals, are seen more as scientists than as healers. Results are what counts with patients. This transformation for physicians has been accelerated by a desire to communicate with the public at large.

Doctors everywhere finally recognize that people are concerned with understanding what is wrong with them and the treatments they receive. The role of the news media cannot be underplayed in this knowledge revolution. Together, organized medicine, through the American Medical Association, along with radio, television, the press, and book publishers, bring information on good health practices to the public.

The length of my medical career is approaching a half-century, and I've seen progress in health and healing. Having received my medical degree way back on June 8, 1952, I chose as my specialty internal medicine, which represented the highest challenge to me. It offered a newly practicing doctor the opportunity to make difficult diagnoses and solve the problems that went along with them. I wanted to be a doctor's doctor, and toward that end, I pursued postgraduate training, not only in internal medicine, but also in pulmonary disease and what I considered to be the pinnacle of diagnostic medicine, cardiology. I've subsequently fulfilled my goals and experienced a satisfying career in diagnostic medicine and cardiology.

Witnessing and participating in the phenomenal changes resulting from new techniques of diagnosis and therapeutics, my colleagues and I have ridden the chariots of challenges. Medical practice has moved from reading simple x-rays to using highly complex diagnostic tools, such as CT scans, MRIs, endoscopies, and fiber optics, all of which improve diagnostic capabilities.

In the field of surgery, we have seen developments which serve not only to minimize patient discomforts but also to reduce their recuperation times. Occasionally, in fact, I regret that today's medical graduates have not been able to witness with me the progress taking place during the last forty-five years.

My impression is that no advance in medicine can compare to those made in the application of antibiotics for overcoming all types of infections. For decades we had been winning the war with microbes. But alas, no more. The widespread implementation of these very antibiotics has created a monstrous world of yeast infections, antibiotic-resistant microorganisms, and persistent, adverse, antibiotic side effects. We in medicine can be faulted for these results.

Today's medical graduates are trained to be skillful in diagnosis. Unfortunately, because of other compelling factors, they must now rely on third parties—the laboratories—to confirm their diagnoses. At the same time, other influences promulgate numerous choices of therapeutic agents—some good and others not so good. Such a scenario has proven detrimental to the patient. The excessive use of synthetic drugs pushed on doctors by the pharmaceutical industry is not a happy circumstance for anyone (except perhaps for the drug companies).

Seeing this begin to happen in my own practice, I began to appreciate the more basic therapeutic agents, long available from mother nature. An open-mindedness to alternatives was required. I changed old treatment habits. My long-held conviction that there is value in complementary medicine led me to embrace avenues of natural treatment.

Soon my medical world opened up. It was a pleasure to experiment with natural and nontoxic remedies. Suddenly I sensed that I now held better tools for accomplishing my mission in medicine, the alleviation of suffering.

Olive leaf extract has shown itself to be among the most significant of these newly uncovered natural, nontoxic therapies. As you'll discover reading this book, olive leaves go beyond the worth of the olive tree's fruit and oil. Olive leaf extract has proven itself to be one of the most important antimicrobials ever discovered.

On these pages, Morton Walker leads us to the next advance in the fight against infectious diseases. Dr. Walker's fascinating tale about the therapeutic applications of olive leaf extract will carry you into areas of health care previously only dreamed of. Carefully researched, Dr. Walker's book documents successful treatment for all kinds of infections arising from fungi, viruses, bacteria, parasites, and other microscopic invaders.

What Dr. Walker is reporting has been my practice experience as well. I have had the privilege of using olive leaf extract on over one hundred patients for the treatment of infections, psoriasis, inflammatory arthritis, and fibrocytis. The results, while not a 100 percent cure rate, have been so much better than what might have been expected that I'm truly enthusiastic about olive leaf extract as potent antimicrobial therapy. My patients are really happy to see me use a natural product rather than a prescribed, synthetic chemical substance, and this natural substance works remarkably well.

So here's a bit of advice: Ride the olive leaf as though it is your magic carpet to better healing and greater health. Know that for thousands of years, people living around the Mediterranean sea have chewed on olive leaves, drunk olive leaf tea, or taken potions made from their tincture as healing agents for really serious problems. Use the miracles described by Dr. Morton Walker, and help your loved ones and yourself.

—Joseph J. Territo, M.D.
Elmwood Park, New Jersey

Preface

In my role as a medical journalist specializing in wholistic health care subjects, I came across this ancient but newly appreciated natural remedy that inhibits or kills microorganisms. I was drawn to the information concerning olive leaf extract in three particular ways. First, the renowned nutritional product developer, Stephen A. Levine, Ph.D., made me aware of oleuropein, the olive tree's main therapeutic ingredient containing potentially useful antimicrobial traits. Second, I long ago recognized the beneficial characteristics of products from the olive tree, having studied the Mediterranean diet which includes olives and their oil. Also, I personally enjoy eating green, golden, and black olives, plus using olive oil for cooking, as a spread on bread, and as part of my salad dressing.

The International Olive Oil Council (IOOC), an intergovernmental agency with twenty-three member states located in Madrid, Spain, has done massive amounts of research on olive oil. However, the IOOC has also discovered numerous benefits accruing to mankind from cultivating the olive tree, not just for its green or golden or black olives, but also for its leaves. Affirmed just last year is that the tree's olive green leaves may be even more advantageous for ingestion than the olive fruit and its oil.

More than any other article I've written for the wholistic medical magazine, the *Townsend Letter for Doctors & Patients,* my column, "Antimicrobial Attributes of Olive Leaf Extract," brought me massive numbers of responses from readers. It appeared in No. 156, the July 1996 issue of that magazine. Queries took the form of over 1,500 telephone calls, letters, e-mails, and faxes (and they're still coming in). For two weeks I was fully occupied responding to inquiries about how olive leaf extract works against microorganisms and where to get it. This spurred me to investigate the subject further and, ultimately, to produce this book.

As recently as early last year, the therapeutic ingredient in olive leaves had been the bane of the olive oil industry, as you'll see. But now those same components are being used to save human beings (and animals) from microbial infections of all kinds. Olive leaf extract kills germs. The active agents, elenolic acid with its salt compound calcium elenolate, are preventatives against colds, flu, the mumps, plus vast numbers of other infections. And they're treatment for them too, if you do come down with any of these infections.

The processed powdered ingredients of olive leaves are extracted and combined into a single, easy-to-swallow capsule. Having come upon olive leaf extract's efficacy as both a preventative and treatment of infection, my wife Joan and myself take the product prophylactically. As a daily supplement to the diet, olive leaf extract can help achieve and maintain the highest levels of good health.

—Dr. Morton Walker
Stamford, Connecticut

Introduction

Residents of Western industrialized countries are currently confronting attacks of pathological "superbug" invaders. Because of immune system degradation among masses of the populace, we are suffering from often inexplicable afflictions brought on by certain ubiquitous disease-producing microorganisms. They are pandemic! Such organisms include:

1. Viruses such as Epstein-Barr and cytomegalovirus, but most especially the retroviruses, such as human immunodeficiency virus (HIV), which don't merely pass through cell membranes but rather take control of the affected cell's genetic machinery.
2. Antibiotic-resistant bacteria, which in some cases actually thrive on the synthetic drugs developed by pharmaceutical companies to kill and/or suppress them.
3. Yeasts and other opportunistic fungi which produce canditoxin and other microtoxins largely responsible for those collective symptoms designated as the yeast syndrome (candidiasis) and chronic fatigue syndrome.

4. Parasites, both as protozoa and helminthic worms, which are the sources of serious diarrheal diseases and constitute the greatest single cause of sickness (morbidity) and death (mortality) for humankind.

Such pathological organisms are associated with (a) an overburdened immune system, (b) the variable diseases of overindustrialization, (c) a deterioration of nature's ecological balance, and (d) the inability of most people to adapt to life amid the changes wrought by high technology.

In such situations, human immunological defenses become so weakened that retroviruses often come out of their dormancy, where they've rested in commensalism. (*Commensalism* is the neutral state in which an organism lives on or in another of a different species without harming or benefiting the host.) When retroviruses such as the Ebola Sudan virus and the Ebola Zaire virus, already present, are awakened to activity by some change, they may readily take hold of their immediate environment by creating pathology within the host's cellular structures.

No single treatment was known to work against any of the superpotent microbial invaders—viruses, antibiotic-resistant bacteria, yeasts, fungi, protozoa, worms—until now. This book discusses a newly discovered antimicrobial agent which actually has been available to mankind since the creation of Genesis in the Bible's Old Testament. It's now in a new, orally administered gelatin capsule containing grayish/brownish/greenish powder which contains an extract of leaves harvested from "the tree of life"—the olive tree, botanically classified as *Olea europaea L.*

Two Million Americans Get Hospital-Acquired Infections

It has been established by scientists studying at the University of Texas Health Science Center at Dallas that over two million residents of the United States enter hospitals each year with one ailment and wind up with another. The mere fact of being in a hospital exposes them to "nosocomial," or hospital-acquired, infections, which are fatal to as many as 22,000 Americans a year and untold numbers in other countries.

"The very technology that saves patients' lives now sets them up for infection," says Robert Haley, M.D., head of the Epidemiology and Preventive Medicine Unit at the University of Texas Health Science Center. "Ten years ago many of these patients would have died, but the techniques that save them bring a risk of infection. We have more burn units, more ICUs [intensive care units], more catheters, more respirators. Every piece of equipment, every invasive technique provides the opportunity for infection to develop."

Worse, antibiotic-resistant organisms are an integral risk of any infection whether they are the original cause of illness or acquired nosocomially. "About the time the cost-price of an antibiotic comes down, the bacterium's resistance to it goes up," Dr. Haley said in a University of Texas press conference.

After forty years of pushing antibiotics for any reason, minor or major, physicians are now confronting bacteria that have mutated and built defenses against drugs. The infectious bacteria have become "superbugs," causing the deaths of patients who succumb to once treatable invasions of these pathological organisms.

How Antibiotics Acted Against Bacteria

Without question, the primary reason for reappearances of highly infectious bacteria (and many other pathogenic microorganisms) cloaked in superresistant mantles lies with conventionally practiced allopathic medicine's overuse and misuse of antibiotics and other drugs. Out of fairness, however, I must mention that a few types of bacteria return with a vengeance because of the ingenious biochemistry of the microorganisms themselves.

Bacteria bring about pathology in particular ways. For a bacterium to cause an infection, it must enter the body and find a place to multiply in large numbers before the body's natural defenses remove it. If the bacterial quantities increase beyond the capability of a person's immune defense system, dire consequences result. As their numbers escalate into the billions, the bacteria bring about illness by churning out microtoxins or by digesting tissues.

In 1928, however, Dr. Alexander Fleming gave the world penicillin, and a new set of therapeutic principles using antibiotics was born. Most antibiotics worked by killing the growing bacterial colony by one of three means:

1. A large number of antibiotics, including penicillin, interfered with the microbe's ability to build its cell wall.
2. Other antibiotics, such as erythromycin and tetracycline, gummed up the machinery that bacteria use to assemble vital proteins.
3. A third antibiotic type adhered to the bacterial chromosome, effectively shutting down reproduction.[1]

To accomplish any of these tasks, the antibiotic either penetrated the body of the bacterium or fitted like a lock-and-key onto a chemical binding site (a receptor) on its outer membrane or cell wall. Because of the microorganisms' mutations in defense, antibiotics hardly create these therapeutic effects anymore. A bacterium's antibiotic receptors don't form. The superbugs are resistant to almost every type of antibiotic created in the past, and nothing in the future holds much promise.[2]

Bacterial immunological genes are a factor too. The bacteria have returned with a vengeance because they are moving targets. If just one in a population of a billion develops a random gene mutation that allows it to survive an antibiotic attack, it passes this immunity along to its offspring. For example, some of the microbes that first developed an immunity to penicillin did so by altering the shape of the cell wall target to which the drug normally attached. Over the years the pharmaceutical industry responded with more powerful (and more expensive) antibiotics. But the bacteria kept upping the ante by altering their own defenses with immunological genes.[3]

This antibiotic immunity is not entirely the result of chance mutation. The superbugs are able to cooperate with each other to resist the antibiotics by exchanging small, self-copying loops of deoxyribonucleic acid (DNA) called *plasmids*. Plasmids contain supplemental genes that may not be present on a bacterium's main chromosome. In addition, these pathological organisms contain ''jumping genes,'' bits of DNA that pop from one microbe to another.[4] ''Bacteria are not separate populations, but part of a vast, interactive microbial world,'' says Stuart Levy, M.D., of Tufts University.

Typical Antibiotic-Resistant Supermicrobes[5]

Bacteria replicate at blinding speed inside the body of an organism (*in vivo*)—sometimes doubling their population within five minutes. The reproductive process can produce genetic mutations that produce bacterial defenses against a given drug—making an enzyme that splits the penicillin molecule, for instance, so it becomes harmless. The microbes can then quickly pass on their genetic armor to offspring.

Some of these super microbes mutate into a ''multi-drug-resistant'' strain, as in the case of one type of tuberculosis which hit major cities and hospitals in 1992. This strain of *Mycobacterium tuberculosis* becomes immune to several medications simultaneously and causes death in 50 percent of its victims.

Then there is the common staphylococcus which may prove deadly when it contaminates a wound, gets inside the body during surgery, or infects someone in a weakened condition, such as a bedridden hospital patient. Although once killed with penicillin, the staphylococci that breed in hospitals have learned to inactivate almost every antibiotic except vancomycin, an intravenous drug with serious, complicating, adverse side effects such as kidney toxicity and hearing loss. And resistance even to this brutal drug has developed in a related, harmful staphylococcus organism— the enterococci—which infect surgical wounds below the waist.

Two common respiratory infectors, *Haemophilus influenzae* and *Streptococcus pneumoniae,* have emerged as antibiotic-resistant. The standard ear and sinus infections often present in children and adults are usually created by *S. pneumoniae.* Both of these infectors can cause meningitis.

According to the United States Centers for Disease Control and Prevention (CDC) in Atlanta, Georgia, cases of food-borne, drug-resistant salmonella have risen from 16 percent of total cases in 1979 to 32 percent in 1989 and 44 percent today.

Even with the thirty or so antibiotics the established pharmaceutical industry claims to be working on, there aren't currently any potent antibiotics left to treat these drug-resistant bacteria. Whatever the companies come up with, all the antibiotics are derived from molds and bacteria in the soil and work through the same narrow mechanisms. Get infected with one of the superresistant pathological organisms, and the odds are that you or your loved one could become exceedingly ill—perhaps die.

For this and other reasons, we need a new, natural, safe, and nontoxic food supplement that's proven itself repeatedly as a means of counteracting invasions of immune-suppressing pathological organisms. The required supplement exists—olive leaf extract—as a readily available item sold by mail order or in health food stores as an over-the-counter, nonprescription product. It's just recently become available for purchase in pharmacies.

Provided here is a full disclosure of the antimicrobial attributes of this newly discovered, generic food supplement which has been growing on earth at least since the time of Noah's ark. Olive leaf extract is society's newest best hope to save itself from being overwhelmed by sexually transmitted diseases, all types of resistant bacteria, overburdening body yeasts, parasites in our drinking water, fungi in gyms and locker rooms, plus Ebola, HIV, and other emerging viruses that outright kill. Thus, this book offers consumers knowledge to protect themselves against current and coming plagues.

The Olive Tree of Life

Right up there with the domesticated dog, the olive tree ranks among man's best friends. For at least 6,000 years, the olive tree's special gifts to humankind have been documented—in the Bible, it's called "the tree of life." An olive branch is the United Nations' global symbol of peace and, as you'll see, it's a symbol of health as well.

The olive tree belongs to a plant family that includes the ash, jasmine, and lilac. Today it's widely cultivated throughout areas surrounding the Mediterranean sea, the source of over 98 percent of the earth's olive oil. A superior tree species, from which olive leaf extract is made, the *Olea europaea L.*, grows in Southern California.

Olive wood, being hard and variegated, is valued in cabinetry.

When Moses was atop Mt. Sinai, the divine recipe for making holy anointing oil included myrrh, cinnamon, aromatic cane, and of course, olive oil.

Greek mythology attributes the creation of olive trees to the goddess Athena, who first planted one among the rocks of the Acropolis. She endowed it with powers to illuminate the darkness, soothe wounds, restore libido, heal illness, and provide nourishment.

For over 2,000 years, olive cultivation, oil and olive curing, and oil production have advanced to become a fine art. The Roman Empire's recipes for using olives and olive oil in food are still used today.

Olive oil illuminated houses along the Mediterranean well into the nineteenth century. It lubricated the machines of the industrial revolution just as it once served the Roman legions as axle grease.

Folk medicines include olive oil as the main ingredient for a variety of afflictions. For example:

- Olive oil mixed with an equal part of limewater is good for burns.
- Olive oil soothes the discomforts of infant teething and inflammations of mucous membranes.
- Hippocrates recommended olive oil for curing ulcers, cholera, and muscular pains.

Olive oil, a monounsaturated fat, is proven by modern allopathic medicine to lower the blood's low-density lipoproteins (LDLs). Many clinical studies point to the consumption of olive oil by Mediterranean peoples as the major reason why they have a lower incidence of heart disease than do Americans.

As you will learn in Chapter 8, on acquired immune deficiency syndrome (AIDS), olive leaf extract combined in a drink of whole lemon, olive oil, and some other substances, turns a person with AIDS (PWA) from being human immunodeficiency virus–positive (HIV-positive) to HIV-negative. Drinking tea brewed from olive leaves works in the same manner as well.[6]

PART ONE

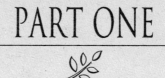

The Developmental History of the Therapeutic Attributes of Olive Leaf Extract

CHAPTER 1

❧

We Swim in a Sea of Microbes

In 1969, the Surgeon General of the United States, William Stewart, declared in a speech to the nation, "The war against infectious diseases has been won." Dr. Stewart was dead wrong!

Probably because he and his advisers failed to recognize the unsustainable efficacy of antibiotics and the powerful mutational characteristics of microbes, what the Surgeon General said has proven to be totally untrue. His statement is even more erroneous today, twenty-eight years later. Now we are faced with new and highly potent germs plus the return of organisms we had believed were conquered, but currently may be considered drug-resistant "superbugs." The golden age of antibiotics has ended.

While the numbers of illnesses and deaths arising from communicable diseases have lessened for people living in the developed, Western, industrialized nations, the balance of our world, especially populations residing in undeveloped countries, suffer constantly from invading microbes. Microbial infections are the primary sources of sicknesses for these people. Virulent diseases have never ceased to be the leading cause of death in poor countries, particularly for young children and the elderly.

Moreover, in North America and throughout Western Europe, just during the 1980s, acquired immunodeficiency syndrome (AIDS), several forms of herpes, chlamydia, and Lyme disease have all appeared as new debilitating disorders. We've witnessed the return of staph infections, measles, syphilis, gonorrhea, septicemia (blood poisoning), bacterial pneumonia, and tuberculosis, old-time diseases thought suppressed beyond resurgence. Once again we face a conflict for dominance between human beings and our microbial enemies.[1]

"All animals coexist with an indigenous microflora. We are each heavily colonized by, and live in a state of peaceful co-existence with, countless microorganisms that colonize our skin and most of our mucosal surfaces," says Stanford T. Shulman, M.D., Chief of the Division of Infectious Diseases at The Children's Memorial Hospital in Chicago. Beginning shortly after birth, "we swim in a veritable sea of microbes," Dr. Shulman adds.[2]

Confirming these comments, Robert J. Herceg, M.D., Resident in Pathology at Northwestern University Medical School in Chicago, and Lance R. Peterson, M.D., Professor of Medicine and Pathology, also at Northwestern University Medical School, join in stating, "The human body is populated by an immense variety of microbial tenants. . . . By various mechanisms that are only beginning to be understood, they interact with each other, with the host, and with potential invading organisms. They are sometimes beneficial in terms of protecting us from outside pathogens, but at times can be harmful, overgrowing and damaging their host."[3]

Despite improved methods of treating and preventing infection such as once-potent antibiotics, rigorous immunizations, and modern methods of sanitation, infection still accounts for much serious illness, even in highly industrialized nations. In third world countries, contagion from infecting microorganisms remains the most pressing of all health problems.[4]

The Medical Specialty of Infectious Diseases

Because disease-producing microorganisms such as bacteria, spirochettes (a type of bacteria), viruses, rickettsiae (bacteria-like parasites), chlamydiae (virus-like bacteria), fungi, yeasts and molds (two specific forms of fungi), protozoa (single-cell animal parasites), helminths (worms), and even algae (primitive plants) cause illnesses, the specialty of infectious diseases has become a clinical division of medicine. Physicians practicing this specialty are concerned with the pathogenesis, diagnosis, and management of sickness directly caused by virulent microbes.

A main thrust of the infectious disease specialist's interest is *epidemiology,* the study of various factors as they relate to the occurrence, frequency, and distribution of disease in a given population. The study of epidemiology includes the origin of the disease, how it's transmitted, and host and environmental influences on the development of disease.

In a situation when an *epidemic* is said to exist, the infectious disease is occurring in the region's population at some level that is higher than normal.

However, an *outbreak* is different. It's a sudden appearance of the disease, often in only a small portion of the area's population.

An *endemic* disease is persistently present in a given locale; a *hyperendemic* disease is persistent also, but it has a high incidence of occurrence among the affected population.

When the infectious disease specialist speaks of a *reservoir,* he or she is referring to the natural habitat of the microorganism responsible for the disease.

The illness may be transmitted from a *source* in which

the infecting organism multiplies more or less extensively. There are various sources, a few more common than others.

Sources which carry a disease between two or more human hosts, such as an animal (the mule deer) or an insect (a deer tick of the genus, *Ixodes,* carrying the infecting spirochete, *Borrelia burghdorferi,* of Lyme disease), are considered *vectors.* People who are infected with a disease or were recently exposed to it are often sources as well (as happens in sexually transmitted diseases).

Disease transmission may also take place through a *vehicle,* like contaminated food or water. Infectious organisms carried in a particular vehicle can multiply within it.[5]

Kinds of Infections to Which We Become Exposed

The invasion and multiplication of microbes in or on body tissues, producing symptoms as well as an immune response, is considered to be an *infection.* In the presence of such an infection, the host (a human being or another animal) is injured by cellular damage from the microorganism's toxins, by its intracellular multiplication, or by the germ's interference with the host's metabolism.

Sometimes the host's own immune response may compound the tissue damage, as in an allergy. The damage may be systemic and spread throughout the body or localized, as occurs in infected pressure ulcers. The infection's severity varies with the virulence (pathogenicity) and number of the invading microorganisms, and the strength of host defenses.

We are exposed to various kinds of infections. For example, when an infection is verified by laboratory investigation but no signs and symptoms show up, the doctor will likely label it a *subclinical, silent,* or *asymptomatic infection.* Added to this is *colonization,* in which the multiplication of microbes produces no signs, symptoms, or immune responses. Then the person with a subclinical infection may become a carrier and transmit the infection to others. Such transmission often happens when someone carries flu germs without showing signs of its presence and then kisses or even shakes hands with another person (colds and flu are spread this way). Personal contact is the cause of much infectious transmission.

A *latent infection* occurs after a microorganism has been dormant in the host, sometimes for years. One will see this frequently when root canal dentistry is performed by endodontists. An endodontist's failure to clean out and disinfect the base of a retained tooth that no longer possesses a viable root can lead to osteitis of the patient's jaw bone years later.

An *exogenous infection* results from environmental pathogens; an *endogenous infection* comes from the host's normal flora, the organisms that permanently—and usually harmlessly—reside within us.[6] In late January 1997, I learned of an endogenous infection striking a seven-month-old baby girl. She acquired a bacterial infection of *Escherichia coli* from her own large intestine. This *E. coli* microbe had been displaced from its usual place of residence in the colon by a blockage in her gut, causing penetration through the walls of her urinary tract. She developed a high fever and for some time was quite sick. Hospitalized, she was treated with Vancomycin, the only antibiotic still effective against E. Coli, and overcame her endogenous infection.

The Microbes That Bring Us Diseases[7]

A *microorganism* or *microbe* is defined as any living thing too small to be visible to the naked eye, most often made up of a single cell. As mentioned above, microbes are classified into *species:* bacteria, spirochetes, viruses, rickettsiae, chlamydiae, fungi, yeasts, molds, protozoa, and helminths. A species is the narrowest such classification. Members of the same species are able to interbreed and produce fertile offspring.

Bacteria are single-cell microorganisms with well-defined cell walls and the ability to multiply independently on artificial media without the need for other cells. In developing countries, where poor sanitation heightens the risk of infection, bacterial diseases commonly cause death and disability. Even in industrialized countries, they're still sources of the most common fatal infectious diseases.

Bacteria can be classified by shape. Spherical bacterial cells are called *cocci;* rod-shaped bacteria, *bacilli;* and spiral-shaped bacteria, *spirilla.* Bacteria can also be classified in four other ways: by (1) their response to staining with dyes (gram-positive, gram-negative, or acid-fast bacteria), (2) their motility, or ability to move, (motile or nonmotile bacteria), (3) their tendency to enclose themselves with a membraneous capsule (encapsulated or nonencapsulated bacteria), and (4) their oxygen requirements (aerobic bacteria require oxygen to grow; anaerobic bacteria do not).

Spirochetes, classified as a type of bacteria, are flexible, slender, undulating spiral rods with cell walls. Most are anaerobic. The three forms of spirochetes pathogenic in humans include *Treponema, Leptospira,* and *Borrelia.*

Rickettsiae are relatively uncommon on the North American continent. They are small, gram-negative, bacteria-like organisms frequently inducing life-threatening infections. Three genera of rickettsiae include *Richettsia, Coxiella,* and *Rochalimaea.*

Viruses are subcellular organisms made up of only a ribonucleic acid (RNA) or a deoxyribonucleic acid (DNA) nucleus covered with proteins. They are the smallest known organisms, so tiny that they're visible only through an electron microscope. Viruses can't replicate independent of host cells. Rather, they invade a host cell and stimulate it to participate in the formation of additional virus particles. The estimated 400 viruses that infect humans are classified according to their size, shape (spherical, rod-shaped, or cubic), or means of transmission (by respiratory, fecal, oral, or sexual routes).

Chlamydiae, classified somewhere between viruses and bacteria, are larger than viruses and were found recently to be intracellular obligate (restricted to a host) bacteria. Unlike other bacteria, they depend on host cells for replication; unlike other viruses, they're susceptible to antibiotics.

Fungi are single-cell organisms with nuclei enveloped by their nuclear membranes. They have rigid cell walls like plant cells but lack chlorophyll, the green matter necessary for photosynthesis. They also show relatively little cellular specialization. Fungi occur as yeasts or molds. Depending on the environment, some fungi may occur in both forms. Fungal diseases in humans are called *mycoses.*

Yeasts, classified as fungi, are single-celled, oval-shaped microorganisms that reproduce both asexually, by budding, and sexually, by the formation of spores. They ferment carbohydrates, producing alcohol and carbon dioxide. Yeast organisms produce germ tubes which grow into human or animal tissues. The germ tubes, known as *mycelia,* are filamentous, thread-like structures that the yeast puts out in search of nutrients for the organism. Tangled masses can develop when local growth conditions change and large numbers of budding yeast suddenly decide to "move out" by forming mycelia. The yeast syndrome, also known as *candidiasis,* a fungal disease which will be discussed in Chapter 11, occurs from the overgrowth of one particular yeast, *Candida albicans.*[8]

Molds are any multicellular filamentous fungus that commonly forms a rough furry coating on decaying matter. As pathological organisms, however, they generally create circular colonies in the host tissues which may appear cottony, woolly, or glabrous, but whose filaments are not organized into large fruiting bodies, such as mushrooms (which are fungi).

Protozoa are the simplest single-cell organisms of the

animal kingdom, but they show a high level of cellular specialization. Like other animal cells, they develop cell membranes rather than cell walls, and their nuclei are surrounded by nuclear membranes.

Helminths are three groups of worm-like creatures that invade humans; they include nematodes, cestodes, and trematodes.

Nematodes are cylindrical, unsegmented, elongated helminths that taper at each end; this shape has earned them the designation *roundworm*.

Cestodes are better known as *tapeworms* and possess bodies that are flattened front to back with distinct, regular segments. Tapeworms also have heads with suckers or sucking grooves.

Trematodes have flattened, unsegmented bodies. They are flukes classified as *blood, intestinal, lung,* or *liver flukes,* depending on their infection site.

We Have Entered the Post-antibiotic Era

Even though the last one hundred years witnessed tremendous advances in the understanding of infectious disease, as we enter the twenty-first century many problems continue. The natural ebb and flow of infection changes almost daily. Moreover, the speed of air travel is such that pathological organisms can readily invade from distant lands. The elimination of one infectious disease highlights another, and the delicate balance prevailing between human beings and microbes remains. Today medical scientists willing to face reality know that there is no final victory over infection, and they accept that the healing professions have entered the post-antibiotic era.[9]

"In their eagerness to finish off the old diseases, doctors and patients have, paradoxically, given them new life," states *Newsweek* magazine.[10] When patients demand antibiotics for a minor viral infection, like a cold or flu, every dose of the drug makes it easier for resistance of microorganisms to grow. Also, physicians occasionally dispense antibiotics without knowing whether a sore throat, or even the symptoms of pneumonia, are indeed caused by bacteria; viral pneumonia is as common a pathological entity as bacterial pneumonia.

When a strain of bacteria such as *Streptococcus pneumoniae* (which produces the pneumonia infection) is treated with any of the penicillins, most of the infecting colony dies. But a few of the invading streptococcus microorganisms, harboring mutant, resistant genes, will survive. Those remaining microbes stay immunologically resistant to the penicillin drugs thereafter.

The mutants pass on their resistance genes to their progeny—and a single bacterium can produce 16,777,220 offspring within twenty-four hours. These newly hatched microbes become the superbugs against which no antibiotic is effective.

The mutants share their resistance genes even with unrelated microbes. For example, cholera bacteria were observed by bacteriologists to have picked up resistance genes to tetracycline from *E. coli,* the common bacteria present in everyone's gastrointestinal tract. Such a mutant gene transfer is accomplished with a chemical exuded to other germs by the mutated bacterium. Using its exuded chemical, the altered superbug draws in a fellow pathogen; when the two touch, they open pores and exchange a loop of DNA called a *plasmid.* This plasmid is an additional chromosomal genetic element that remains stable and functions or replicates while physically separate from the chromosome of the bacterial host cell. It is not essential to the cell's basic functioning. As a result of such plasmid transfer, a number of drug-resistant microbes have developed in human beings, including enterococcus, haemophilus influenzae, mycobacterium tuberculosis, neisseria gonorrhoeae, plasmodium falciparum, shigella dysenteriae, staphylococcus aureus, and streptococcus pneumoniae. Dozens of the drugs we've used, including penicillins, tetracycline, and ampicillin, have been removed from our arsenal of weapons against specific diseases.

The treatment of diseases caused by viruses presents another set of complex problems. Few drugs can be developed as antiviral products because of the microbe's nature. Because viruses are parasites that exist within living cells, it is difficult to manufacture any type of pharmaceutical agent that will kill the virus without killing the human host cell in which it is lodged. That's why the pharmaceutical industry has developed almost no antiviral medicines; those they have are mainly used to treat very sick hospitalized patients or people with deficient immune systems. Until the development of olive leaf extract as a virucide, we had to rely almost entirely on our immune systems to fight viral infections.[11]

As you're about to learn, this is not the situation anymore. Circumstances have changed. There is a new and natural food supplement which, with nature-made medicines, synthetic drugs, or other treatment utilized by doctors, can help those millions of people who are victims of a compromised immune system. Because drug-resistant bacteria and other pathological microbes have arisen during recent decades, olive leaf extract has became a vital food supplement.

Olive Leaf Extract Kills Viruses, Bacteria, Fungi, and Parasites

There's a need for a natural, readily obtainable antiviral agent that does no damage to human cells but acts as a virucide against the pathogenic organisms that cause viral diseases such as hepatitis, herpes simplex, flu, Epstein-Barr, and the common cold. Such a therapeutic agent exists, of course—it has been growing on olive trees for four to six thousand years but has been largely overlooked by Western medicine. The powdered extract of olive leaves kills not only viruses but most every other type of disease-producing microorganism.

Olive leaf extract is an antifungal agent. It obliterates fungal, yeast, or mold infestations such as athlete's foot, ringworm, thrush, vaginal yeast infections, and many other disorders that arise from microscopic plant invaders.

Olive leaf extract is an antiparasitic as well, killing or driving out other microscopic animals or plants that live in or on the human body. Chemical components of the olive leaf work against various *endoparasites* that thrive inside the body, such as two particular organisms offered here as examples, the amoeba *Entamoeba histolytica* and the protozoa *Giardia lamblia*.[12] The same olive leaf components eliminate *ectoparasites,* tiny animals which live on the body's surface like mites and ticks.

Based on my research, I am convinced that olive leaf extract is destined to become the most useful, wide spectrum, antimicrobial herbal ingredient of the twenty-first century. As you read further, you'll come to understand the reasons for my enthusiasm.

As early as 1948, that great microbiologist René J. Dubos, Ph.D., of The Rockefeller Institute for Medical Research in New York City, explained the mechanisms through which harmful microbes reach their potential victims and elicit pathologic reactions. He didn't see the sense of attacking microorganisms so aggressively at the expense of the human host. Dr. Dubos cited the need to explore how and why microorganisms and human cells often remain in a state of peaceful coexistence. He could have been making the case for olive leaf extract as an antimicrobial agent. Here is what Dr. Dubos wrote:

Aggressive warfare against microbes has been the ortho-dox approach of medical microbiology to the problems of disease, and it is obvious that this policy has made and is still making immense contributions to the improvement of health. But it is also increasingly apparent that without benefit of drugs or vaccines, the majority of human beings, as well as of animals and plants, commonly reach a state of equilibrium with even the most virulent pathogens. In the normal course of events, all sorts of microorganisms become established and persist in the tissues without interfering with the normal physiologic processes of their hosts—a condition that one might call peaceful coexistence. The very fact that infection need not result in disease, and indeed rarely does, suggests that aggressive warfare against pathogens may not be the only profitable approach of medical microbiology to the maintenance of health; it points to the possibility that techniques could be developed for rendering the body capable of converting parasitism into commensalism. [13]

As you will recognize from the balance of this book, olive leaf extract complies with the concept put forth by Dr. René Dubos fifty years ago. Finally, medical science has found the means to neutralize most kinds of pathological microorganisms, not with any sort of drug, but with a nonprescription, over-the-counter food supplement.

CHAPTER 2

✌

The Development of Olive Leaf Extract as an Antimicrobial Agent

Between 1827 and 1855, medical information appeared describing the bitter tea brewed from leaves of the olive tree (*Olea europaea*) as a potential cure of the protozoa-caused disease, malaria. Olive leaves were boiled in water and the solution was administered as a drink to malaria patients. Sometimes it was mixed with wine to make a drink called *Tinctura Olea Foliorum*. Dispensed that way, the antimalarial components in olive leaves were being presented as an aqueous extract turned into a hydroethanolic extract. Doctors' reports of patients' improvement came out of these trials but were not acted upon by health professionals until recently.

To illustrate how old medical information is being put to modern use, let me insert just one instance. A chiropractor with an affinity for nutritional research, Bern Friedlander, of San Mateo, California, is using olive leaf extract for therapeutic purposes against malaria. Since tablets or capsules containing the powdered extract of olive leaves are proven to exhibit an antiprotozoan effect, Dr. Friedlander, whom I shall discuss further in Chapter 6, is engaged in a study of 100 Taiwanese people suffering from malaria. Dr.

Friedlander is supervising the dispensing of olive leaf compound by Taiwanese physicians to their malaria patients. The modern, nondrug, medical use of olive leaf extract against this parasitic disease is so "different" and encouraging, results won't be ready for reporting until they are verified by a placebo-controlled, double-blind study of the 100 patients. This report should be issued sometime next year.

Farther into the nineteenth century, more careful basic research was carried out by biochemists on powdered olive leaves. They analyzed the leaf matrix and determined that it is a phenolic compound, which they gave the Latin name *oleuropein*. It was isolated from the olive leaf and considered to be the source of the olive tree's powerful disease-resistant properties. Several separate laboratory evaluations have shown oleuropein to be a bitter glucoside present in the pulp of olive fruits.[1]

Chemically, glucoside is one of a group of compounds containing the cyclic forms of glucose (a sugar), in which the hydrogen of the hemiacetal hydroxyl radical in the compound's chemical ring has been replaced by an alkyl or aryl group. Then, according to botanists, oleuropein, which is present throughout the olive tree—in its wood, fruit, leaves, roots, and bark—helps to protect the tree against insect and bacterial predators.[2]

Some of the pests attempting to attack olive trees occasionally do succeed, but most of the time this natural pesticide, oleuropein, fights off the attackers. The everpresent pests consist of: (1) the lacy-winged olive fly, *Dacus oleae,* which tries to deposit eggs into olives, sometimes causing the fruit to drop off or acquire a wormy-tasting oil; (2) the black scale of *Coccus oleae,* which occasionally clings to leaves on the bark and attracts another pest, (3) a fungus called *fumagine;* (4) tuberculosis tumors and a few other diseases; (5) borers of different types; (6) moths; and (7) spiders. All of these pests are counteracted rather effectively by the olive trees' oleuropein.[3]

By 1969, more molecular analyses had taken place and the main antimicrobial ingredient present in oleuropein was uncovered by researchers at The Upjohn Company of Kalamazoo, Michigan. Inhibiting the growth of every virus, bacterium, fungus, yeast, and protozoon that it was tested against, this antimicrobial ingredient was identified as the calcium salt of elenolic acid, marked in chemistry as *calcium elenolate.*

The Upjohn Company, a giant corporation in the pharmaceutical industry, assigned its scientists to investigate calcium elenolate in order to introduce it to the marketplace as a patented new drug. They were especially anxious to develop oleuropein's calcium elenolate component into a virucide because there weren't any protected by patent and available for sale at the time. (Even today there are almost no virucides patented and available.) From testing on agar medium in petridishes (*in vitro*) and in laboratory animals *(in vivo),* the Upjohn scientists found that viruses which were killed by the olive leaf substance are the coxsackievirus, the parainfluenza 3 virus, the herpesvirus, the pseudorabies virus, the vesicular stomatitis virus, the encephalomyocarditis virus, Newcastle disease virus, poliovirus, and the Sindbis virus.[4]

How Olive Leaf Extract Works Against Microbes

Pure calcium elenolate is obtained after mild acid hydrolysis from the aqueous extracts of various parts of the olive plant. The calcium salt is of crystalline form derived from its hydrolysates.[5] This crystalline substance is powdered for creating tablets or capsules of the virucidal nutritional supplement being dispensed to patients by health care professionals.

In a document describing how it works, James R. Privitera, M.D., of Covina, California, advises that olive leaf extract brings about:

- A critical interference with certain amino acid production processes necessary for the vitality of a specific virus, bacterium, or other microbe.
- Interference with viral infection and/or spread by inactivating viruses or by preventing virus shedding, budding, or assembly at the cell membrane.
- Direct penetration into infected host cells and irreversible inhibition of microbial replication.
- Neutralization of the retrovirus's production of reverse transcriptase as well as protease. (These two enzymes are essential for a retrovirus such as human immunodeficiency virus [HIV] to alter the ribonucleic acid [RNA] of a healthy cell.)
- Direct stimulation of phagocytosis as an immune system response to germs of all types.

Because calcium elenolate was found by The Upjohn Company to rapidly bind to proteins in blood serum and thus be rendered ineffective, the drug company came to a business decision and discontinued developing calcium elenolate as a pathogenic microorganism—killing any pharmaceutical product for commercial distribution in the 1970s. However, by 1994, independent scientific researchers had experimented sufficiently and accomplished a therapeutic breakthrough. It opened the way for clinical application of olive leaf extract as a viable nutritional supplement for all types of antimicrobial use.

The "Die-off" Connected with Olive Leaf Extract

Only one adverse effect comes with use of olive leaf extract: the Herxheimer reaction. Named after the German physician Karl Herxheimer, M.D., the Herxheimer reaction is a "die-off" involving the pathological organisms causing disease. When alive, the harmful microbes seem able to evade the immune system to some degree. But when killed by the olive leaf's therapeutic components, their cell-wall proteins are absorbed through the weakened mucous membrane and cause the patient to experience allergic reactions. Antibodies stimulated by the organisms' infections react at sites in the tissues of present or previous infection.

Thus, "die-off," referred to in medicine as the "Herxheimer reaction," occurs when the olive leaf component kills large numbers of harmful germs rather quickly. Then, the patient's membranes absorb toxic products from these dead microorganisms. The large amount of foreign antigens triggers an increasing immune response, in addition to interfering with usual biochemical processes, and these immune effects can temporarily worsen a person's symptoms. Physicians using olive leaf extract believe that this die-off reaction indicates that the treatment is working. Die-off therefore suggests that the patient is having an excellent response to a properly designed treatment program.[6]

Some of the symptoms of the Herxheimer reaction are due to formation of immune complexes (antigens reacting with antibodies) with resulting histamine release, swelling, and pain. The tissue surfaces where the germ has infected and where histamine reactions are most distressing turn out to be the following areas: mucous membranes in the mouth, esophagus, stomach, small and large intestines, sexual and urinary organs, sinuses, Eustachian tubes in the ears, bronchi, lymphatics, and other membranes such as the meninges (protective wrappings) of the brain and synovial linings of the joints. Any of these locations can be a source of discomfort when die-off takes place. Almost every discomfort connected with die-off disappears within four days to a week.[7] Then the patient who has been taking the olive leaf extract often feels fabulously well—better than ever before.

A nonpracticing naturopathic physician residing in Las

Vegas, Nevada, John Voorhees, N.D., performed a series of experiments using olive leaf extract and various *Lactobacillus* strains, including acidophilus, bulgarus, and caucacius. Dr. Voorhees prepared a single cup batch of soy milk and cows milk for yogurt production, which he incubated at 110°F for twelve hours. To this he added the bacteria-killing powder from one capsule of olive leaf extract. The finished yogurt was unaffected by any ingredient in the antimicrobial agent; instead, it tasted rich and fullbodied, just as is accomplished with any well-prepared yogurt product.

Then Dr. Voorhees repeated the experiment with two capsules of olive leaf extract. At the end of twelve hours, he reports, his yogurt was delicious. The naturopath suggests that anyone can perform this experiment and achieve the same result.

By making yogurt with olive leaf extract as part of the culture, Dr. Voorhees's experiment proves that friendly gut bacteria are not impaired or destroyed by the antimicrobial agent in olive leaf extract. It seems to have an affinity only for pathogens.

Benefits of Taking Olive Leaf Components

Only one method of manufacture exists to produce olive leaf extract that is truly therapeutic. All conventional extraction methods create a powdered concentration whose active ingredients bind rapidly to serum proteins in the blood, rendering them virtually useless in living organisms *(in vivo)*. This problem had thwarted the efforts of researchers for over 100 years. As mentioned above, protein binding of the hydrolysis products of oleuropein in the blood was the problem that caused The Upjohn Company to discontinue development of calcium elenolate as a patented pharmaceutical product. The problem was finally solved in 1995, and while the production process remains proprietary, what can be revealed are the actual olive leaf components which have remedial properties.

First, here is a partial list of the therapeutic benefits provided by taking capsules of olive leaf extract. They are:

- the generalized degradation of pathological microorganisms of all types—viruses, retroviruses, bacteria, spirochetes, rickettsiae, chlamydiae, fungi, yeasts, molds, protozoa, helminths, and other parasites
- the relief of arthritic inflammations, especially osteoarthritis and rheumatoid arthritis
- the reduction of insulin dosages for better control over the risks of symptomatic diabetes
- the elimination of chronic fatigue and the symptoms associated with its syndrome
- the creation or restoration of abundant energy with prolonged stamina
- the normalization of heart beat irregularities (arrhythmias)
- the improvement of blood flow in cardiovascular and/ or peripheral vascular disorders
- the lessening of pain from hemorrhoids
- the attenuation of toothaches
- the antioxidant quenching of free radical pathology
- the obliteration of fungal infections such as mycotic nails, athlete's foot, and jock itch
- the permanent relief of malaria (from a protozoa), dengue fever (from a virus), and other exotic and deadly tropical diseases which produce fever as a primary symptom
- the prevention and effective treatment of all types of viral diseases, including the Epstein-Barr virus, cytomegalovirus, the herpes viruses, human herpes virus-6, the retroviruses, the influenza viruses, viruses of the common cold, and the human immunodeficiency virus (HIV)

- the reversal of almost all symptomatology connected with *Candida albicans* and other organisms causing the yeast syndrome
- the death and excretion of a variety of parasites, including microscopic protozoa and macroscopic helminth worms[8]

Conquering Most Microbe Types with Olive Leaf Extract

An amazing personal case history of conquering most types of microbe classifications by using olive leaf extract was furnished to me by a nutritional counselor in Carmel, California. During a telephone interview I conducted in late August 1996, forty-nine-year-old Melanie Raxford gave me permission to publish her story of ill health and recovery.

Ms. Raxford described how she had experienced the collapse of her immune system about fifteen years before. She came down at that time with chemical sensitivities, allergies, hypothyroidism, and tuberculosis. Then she was struck by a series of opportunistic infections from assorted microorganisms, including candidiasis, Lyme disease, the spuma retrovirus, tularemia, pseudomonas, and other serious health problems such as infestation by protozoa (animal parasites). To define the woman's illnesses:

Lyme disease is a tick-transmitted, spirochetal infection from the bacterium *Borrelia burgdorferi*, which produces acute inflammatory arthritis involving one or more joints.

The spuma form of retroviruses, also known as "foamy" viruses, comes from the subfamily *Spumavirinae*. It exhibits typically persistent, debilitating, flulike symptoms, like those affecting people complaining of "chronic fatigue syndrome," more accurately diagnosed as chronic fatigue and immune dysfunction syndrome (CFIDS).

Tularemia is an infectious disease of animals that shows up in humans as a result of immune suppression. It's caused by the bacillus *Francisella (Pasteurella) tularensis,* which is transmitted by insect carrier or direct contact. It is marked by fever, headache, and open skin sores with localized lymph node enlargement, eye infection, stomach sores, and intestinal sores. The condition is also referred to as *deerfly fever* or *rabbit fever.*

Pseudomonas is a kind of bacteria found in infections of the urinary tract, the ear, and other areas, occurring on and in debilitated patients with diminished immunological resistance. These infections are not treated with antibiotics, but require measures such as the use of 1 percent acetic acid irrigations.

"My body was dying," explained Melanie Raxford. "My lymph nodes were Ping-Pong-ball size. Realizing that I was very toxic, I went on an herbal program and detoxification. I traveled from doctor to doctor looking for help, but so many health professionals were frightened by the numerous illnesses affecting me that usually they declared that nothing much could be done. The spuma virus was nastiest of all, causing me to experience chronic fatigue syndrome among my other problems. There were a great deal of difficulties that I had to overcome, and it was taking years. On my own, I tried some "different" treatments, the electromagnetic frequency generator, homeopathic remedies, and essential oils. These did help quite a bit.

"I was trying to build up my immune system, and then I got lucky by being referred to the use of olive leaf extract. Until I found this concentrate of olive leaves, the longest time I felt somewhat symptom-free was three weeks. After starting on olive leaf extract, I went through nine full weeks without any discomforts from bacteria, viruses, fungi, yeasts, or parasites. Suddenly I had a sense of well-being—like I was nineteen years old again," declared Ms. Raxford. "I took two capsules a day at first and experienced no die-off reaction as sometimes happens. So I went to one capsule, three times per day for several weeks. Eventually I stepped up my dosage to two capsules, three times daily, and have remained at that intake with tremendously beneficial results. Since being on the olive leaf product, all my symptoms are gone. In five months, I haven't undergone any of my prior troubles. I can now count on being functional every day— can make appointments and keep them. It's one of the most exciting times in my life."

Interviewing the woman again during the first week of April 1997, I learned that she was thriving and a bundle of energy. The discomfort of chronic fatigue and immune dysfunction syndrome has long since gone. No disease symptoms have affected Ms. Raxford in any way for over thirty-five weeks. Laboratory examinations of her body fluids and metabolic wastes conducted by the patient's physicians no longer revealed any signs of her prior infections with viruses, bacteria, spirochetes, fungi, yeasts, molds, or parasites. She didn't experience chemical sensitivities, allergies, or hypothyroidism anymore. The acid-fast tuberculosis bacillus, *Mycobacterium tuberculosis,* couldn't be found in her lungs either. The doctors declared her well once again.

"As a nutritional counselor, I've made olive leaf extract available for my clients. Before doing so, I conducted an experiment among six of the people who use my services. All of them reported that olive leaf concentrate has done good things for them," said Ms. Raxford. "They are getting rid of their colds, herpes infections, bacterial infections, and other troubles. It's working phenomenally well for candidiasis and various fungal infections too.

"One of my clients was having intestinal adhesions, throat and lung infection problems, and suffering awfully from severe exhaustion. She took the capsules filled with powdered olive leaf and three weeks later told me, 'My illnesses have disappeared, and I have found energy once again. I can function so much better now.' Why I think that energy develops from the encapsulated olive leaf is that the immune system is being released from wasting itself to conquer all the different types of opportunistic infections. The olive leaf extract does that job efficiently so that energy is left over for a person to feel and function really well. We keep all the energy for our own use and not to fight infections,'' suggested Melanie Raxford.

Facts About Olives

Standing on six continents around the world, an estimated 800 million olive trees cover 24,850,000 acres.

The International Olive Oil Council, a commercial organization concerned with olive tree statistics, says that 90 percent of our planet's olive trees border on the Mediterranean sea. Countries producing most of the olive oil each year are Spain, Italy, France, Sicily, Portugal, Albania, Algeria, Cyprus, Egypt, Israel, Morocco, Tunisia, Turkey, Greece, Yugoslavia, Bulgaria and other Baltic states, and additional European nations. But there are 20 million trees growing in China and another million flourishing in Angola and Zimbabwe. Australia has olive trees growing on its hills, as does New Zealand. And finally, the United States turns out good olive oil (as well as the best olive leaves for extracting into a powder for food supplementation).

While Italy comes to mind when one thinks of olive oil, oil labeled *Italian* often comes from Spain, Greece, Turkey, Morocco, or Tunisia. In fact, Spain cultivates more olive trees than any other country—possibly 50 percent more than Italy. Spain produces about 37 percent of the world's supply, as compared to Italy, which furnishes 19 percent, and Greece 17 percent.

Olive Oil

There are at least seventy-five varieties of olives and olive trees. From them, more than 9,000,000 metric tons of olives are picked annually, with only 800,000 tons packed and consumed as table olives. The rest are turned into soap and oil. Olive oil is a food staple among people living along the Mediterranean, and it's one of the healthier foods available, because it's a monounsaturated fat.

Medical writer and editor Jean Barilla, M.S., in her information-filled book, *Olive Oil Miracle*, says: "Using olive oil in place of saturated fats as the main fat in your diet may actually reduce cholesterol levels. . . . The monounsaturated fats, unlike those in meat and butter, actually promote health. Medical studies are showing that populations that consume lots of monounsaturate-rich olive oil experience remarkable freedom from heart disease and other degenerative conditions."[9]

How Olive Oil Is Graded[10]

Olive Oil is graded by its level of acidity. The "first cold-pressed" oils have the least amount of acidity. Oils from the second, third, and fourth pressings show proportionately much higher acidity.

Extra Virgin Olive Oil is most free of acidity, with an oleic acid content of not more than 1 gram per 100 grams of oil and an organoleptic rating of 6.5 or more. (*Organoleptic* refers to a panel of ten trained tasters who grade the oil from 0 with extremely intense defects to 9 with no defects.) Extra virgin olive oil is least tampered with after its first pressing, plus it has perfect flavor, color, aroma, and no more than 1 percent acidity.

Fine Virgin Olive Oil has an oleic acid content of only 1.5 grams per 100 grams and an organoleptic rating of 5.5 or more.

Semi-fine or Ordinary Virgin Olive Oil has an oleic acid content of not more than 3.3 grams per 100 grams and an organoleptic rating of 3.5 or more.

Lampante Virgin Olive Oil is not fit for consumption unless it undergoes further processing. Lampante means "lamp oil" and is intended for refining or for technical purposes.

Refined Olive Oil, although obtained from virgin olive oils, is unsuitable for consumption because of high acidity or poor flavor. It has poor color, odor, or taste and must be refined.

Olive Oil is a blend of refined olive oil and virgin olive oil. It's no longer labeled "Pure Olive Oil," but its acidity is less than 1.5 grams of oleic acid per 100 grams of oil. The taste is variable.

Olive Pomace Oil is obtained by treating olive pomace with solvents. *Pomace* is the solid part of the olive paste or mash which contains the bulk of the fruit's skin, pulp, and pieces of olive pit (stone), with a certain amount of oil.

Crude Olive-Pomace Oil is intended for food use after refining, or intended for technical purposes. It has poor taste, color, or odor.

Refined Olive-Pomace Oil is intended for consumption as it is or after blending with virgin olive oil.

Olive-Pomace Oil is fit for consumption after blending with refined olive-pomace oil and virgin olive oil, but it cannot be labeled "olive oil."

The Mediterranean Diet

In Greece, every individual, from babies to the very old, consumes an average of five gallons of olive oil each year. The Greeks eat the healthiest diet in the world—the Mediterranean diet. Olive oil is the main cooking oil for the entire Mediterranean region, while other vegetable oils and hydrogenated oils are excluded. At the May 1996 meeting of the American College for Advancement in Medicine in Orlando, Florida, the President of the Center for Genetics, Nutrition and Health, Artemis P. Simopoulos, Ph.D., stated that the ideal diet is based on the traditional diet of people living along the Mediterranean sea. Dr. Simopoulos stated that these ideal foods consisted of olives and olive oil, lemons, vinegar, yogurt, bread, cheese, fruits, nuts, garlic, onions, herbs, spices, pasta, rice, potatoes, poultry, fish, legumes, and other vegetables. They make up the healthiest of all diets.[11]

The majority of these foods with healthful characteristics have been designated by nutritional therapists (doctors who use nutrition instead of drugs for purposes of healing) as being filled with *phytochemicals*, chemical components in plant foods. Such phytochemicals possess a certain quality of *nutriceuticals*—nutrients with pharmaceutical-like actions and no adverse side effects.

The products coming from an olive tree are loaded with beneficial phytochemicals. They offer people nutriceutical properties present not only in its fruit but also packed in the tree's bark, roots, stems, and most of all, its leaves—especially when an antimicrobial extract is made from them.

CHAPTER 3

Uncovering the Therapeutic
Components of Olive Leaf Extract

During the hostilities between Spain and France from 1808 to 1813, Spanish physicians on the front lines of battle made a discovery that was tantamount to unveiling a secret military weapon. They developed a bitter green drink made from ground olive leaves, and administered it as a therapeutic beverage to wounded soldiers suffering from high fevers. This drink brought down the patients' dangerously elevated temperatures from above 104°F to a harmless low-grade level below 101°F. Thus, even feverish Spanish soldiers were able to quickly advance to the fighting ranks once again and push back their French counterparts.

Observing these renewed attacks, by 1811 the French medical corps sent out undercover agents. The military doctors wanted to learn what was happening among the Spaniards. Uncovering the medical secret, the French officer-surgeons quickly adapted the same pulverized green olive leaf drink as part of their own febrifuge (fever-lowering) remedy. The beverage worked so effectively that they prescribed the olive leaf concentrate as a substitute for cinchona bark, which had previously been their standard febrifuge.

Having served in Spain in 1811, Colonel Etiene Pallas,

M.D., of the French Foreign Legion, analyzed the therapeutic ingredients in this olive leaf beverage and eventually published his findings in three separate places: an 1827 book describing his war experiences,[1] an 1828 medical journal article,[2] and in another 1829 volume of his memoirs.[3] Each time, he reported that the olive tree's leaves and young bark contain, among other less important constituents, a crystallizable substance he designated *Vauqueline,* a bitter ingredient to which he ascribes most of the febrifuge properties of the olive tree's plant product.

"Vauqueline," according to Dr. Pallas, "is a colorless, non-odorous solid, having a slightly odd taste. It crystallizes in micaceous [resembling the mineral silicate mica] plates, or sometimes in stellate [star-shaped] prismatic crystals, which are very soluble in water at all temperatures. It scarcely dissolves in cold alcohol, though readily in boiling alcohol, from which it precipitates as the solution cools. Its aqueous solution imparts a faint blue color to reddened litmus paper."

Dr. Pallas also writes: "That some therapeutic value does really attach to the leaves of the olive tree is supported by the fact that both the lilac *(Syringa vulgaris, L.)* and the ash *(Fraxinus excelsior, L.),* plants of the same natural order, are reputed to possess febrifuge properties, and are employed on that account in some parts of the continent."

Dr. Pallas's findings have been ignored by the conventional allopathic medical community until now. The fever-reducing quality of olive leaf extract is but one small (but important) characteristic of its therapeutic components. There are a minimum of one hundred more such characteristics.

These components in olive leaves are not only therapeutically effective as a preventative and treatment for all kinds of health problems but have been proven to be absolutely safe as well. They are projected by biochemists to be as safe for ingestion as purified drinking water, because their toxicity is so low it's practically unmeasurable.

The Safety of Therapeutic Components in Olive Leaf Extract

The newly found phytochemicals in powdered olive leaf extract have undergone toxicity testing and produced no adverse side effects in laboratory animals or in several thousand human subjects.

Oleuropein, the bitter glucoside lodged in the leaves of the green olive tree, and products of its hydrolysis, contain certain components which are valuable as newly discovered therapy for both infectious and degenerative diseases. The empirical formula of oleuropein ($C^{25}H^{32}O^{13}$) makes it a member of the iridoid group, a uniquely structured chemical class which contains a carbohydrate component appearing as D-glucose.

The first iridoid found in nature, *verbenalin,* was isolated as early as 1835, but no investigation into the group's structure began until 1963. That's because iridoids are extremely unstable, and one member of the group has the capability to transform into another. This is the biogenetic characteristic which imparts the unique therapeutic advantages of components within the iridoid oleuropein.[4]

In checking for oleuropein toxicity, doses as high as 1 gram per kilogram (1 g/kg) of body weight for 7 days were used in experiments with mice. The dosage exerted no toxic effects. In fact, oleuropein in olive leaf extract is so safe that the investigators were unable to determine the lethal dose fifty (LD^{50}) or even the toxic dose. The LD^{50} is a calculated dose of any chemical substance which is expected to cause the death of 50 percent of an entire defined experimental animal population, as determined from exposure to the substance.[5]

Most recently it was discovered through scientific investigations that elenolic acid, one of oleuropein's hydrolysis products, is the chief destroyer or growth inhibitor of all kinds of pathological microorganisms. Another hydrolysis product, aglycone, joins elenolic acid in its inhibitory effect. The oleuropein components worked efficiently against those many organisms potentially harmful for humans that are listed in Table 7 of Chapter 10.[6]

As far back as 1969, The Upjohn Company conducted experiments to determine the exact toxicity of a calcium compound derived from elenolic acid, calcium elenolate. Calcium elenolate, a salt, is a potent antimicrobial with the capacity of killing organisms from all species of microscopic growth. Toxicity tests were carried out on laboratory rats, mice, dogs, chickens, and rabbits. In their abstract of the 1970 published report, the researchers wrote:

The LD^{50} of calcium elenolate for rats was approximately 1,700 mg/kg when the drug was administered orally as a single dose [exceedingly safe and nontoxic]. When the drug was given intraperitoneally the LD^{50} was 160 mg/kg in rats and 120 mg/kg in mice [both exceedingly safe and nontoxic]. Daily oral doses of 30, 100, and 300 mg/kg for 30 days were well tolerated in rats [exceedingly safe and nontoxic]. Calcium elenolate was also well tolerated in dogs at 3, 10, and 30 mg/kg per day for 1 month [safe and nontoxic], except for mild gastric irritation at the highest dose tested. The intranasal instillation of 1% and 2% aqueous solutions as drops three times daily in chickens was accompanied by nasal exudation and alterations in the epithelium and lamina propria of the nasal turbinates after 2 days of treatment. Changes in the olfactory epithelium were more pronounced than those in the respiratory epithelium [safe and nontoxic]. Similar though much milder changes were seen in rabbits subjected to aqueous intranasal sprays in concentrations as high as 0.6% four times daily for periods up to 14 days [safe and nontoxic]. Histologically, the reactions of rabbits treated with concentrations of 0.1% and 0.3% were not different from those of control animals after 7 days of treatment; however, the 0.3% concentration when given for 14 days was moderately irritating [safe and nontoxic]. Differences in the distribution of epithelium and total area of the epithelial surface of the human nasal cavity suggest that the rabbit nasal cavity may be more sensitive than that of the human.[7]

As a conclusion to their report, the three authors went further and performed toxicity testing on human volunteers. They affirm that the humans accepted calcium elenolate as a spray applied to their nasal mucosa without any difficulty. Such nose sprays were exceedingly safe, nontoxic, and well tolerated in concentrations of 0.0085 percent to 2 percent. Subsequently, a 1 percent concentration given to the volunteers four times daily was exceedingly safe, nontoxic, and well tolerated for 14 days. That's because human nasal mucosa is less sensitive and reacts less defensively than does rabbit nasal mucosa.[8] This suggests that olive leaf extract would make a highly safe and rather ideal antiviral, over-the-counter nasal spray treatment for people with stuffy noses arising from common colds and the flu (see Chapter 9).

The addition of elenolic acid or its calcium salt, to the germinations of some of the rarer organisms causing disease inhibits them, for instance, *Bacillus cereus* T spores,[9] as well as microfungi, nearly all viruses, most bacteria, and the pathological protein secreted by *Staphylococcus aureus,* which causes almost all hospital-based infections (nosocomial disease).[10]

A Typical Staphylococcus aureus Nosocomial Infection

Gary A. Noskin, M.D., Assistant Professor of Medicine at Northwestern University Medical School, reported on a fifty-five-year-old man whom he admitted to the Northwestern University Hospital in Chicago with substernal chest pain and low blood pressure. The patient was diagnosed as having acute myocardial infarction. Emergency placement of a pulmonary artery catheter and an intraaortic ballon pump was carried out to save his life. Despite a good recovery in the intensive care unit, on the fourth hospital day, the patient developed a fever of 101.5°F associated with chills.

Suspecting bacteremia (generalized blood poisoning) owing to an infected venous catheter, the physician in charge obtained two sets of blood cultures from the patient. The man had been colonized by *Staphylococcus aureus,* and his infection was raging. Not yet knowing about olive leaf extract as an effective antidote for *S. aureus,* Dr. Noskin had no choice but the one remaining antibiotic available, vancomycin. (All other antibiotics fail against antibiotic-resistant organisms like *S. aureus.*) The patient's temperature gradually improved, and he had no more fever (afebrile) within forty-eight hours. After fourteen days of antibiotic therapy, there was no more evidence of metastatic infection or cardiac murmur. Vancomycin was discontinued and the patient underwent coronary angiography and an uncomplicated percutaneous transluminal coronary angioplasty.

Dr. Noskin's patient had undergone the complication of a nosocomial infection, the hospital-acquired microbe invasion that's an increasing problem in the United States, and a major source of illness and death. "The risk of developing an infection while hospitalized in the U.S. is approximately 5 percent. The annual cost of treating these infections is more than $5 billion and significantly increases length of stay, morbidity, and mortality," states Dr. Noskin. "For example, nosocomial bacteremia results in an average increase in hospitalization by 7.4 days at a cost of over $5,000 per episode. The death rate related to nosocomial bloodstream infections is 13.1 percent."[11]

Simply defined, a *nosocomial infection* is one for which there is no evidence that the infection was present or incubating at the time of hospitalization. In general, an infection is considered nosocomial if it occurs more than forty-eight hours after admission to the hospital or occurs in association with frequent outpatient visits to a hospital clinic. Besides the bacterium *S. aureus,* nosocomial infections arise from body invasion of immunosuppressed hospital patients by a great number of other bacteria. They include coagulase-negative staphylococci, vancomycin-resistant enterococci (VRE), aerobic gram-negative bacilli such as *Escherichia coli, Proteus mirabilis, Serratia marcescens, Klebsiella, Enterobacter, Stenotrophomonas maltophilia, Acineto-bacter,* and *Pseudomonas* species.

In addition, nosocomial fungal infections and viral infections can occur during hospitalization. The yeast, *Candida albicans,* is associated with urinary tract infections (UTIs). Cytomegalovirus causes a mononucleosis-like syndrome in normal hospitalized hosts and severe pneumonitis or hepatitis in immunocompromised patients. Hospitalized babies and children not uncommonly come down with nosocomial infections from respiratory syncytial virus, influenza, parainfluenza, adenovirus, rhinovirus, as well as varicella and measles.[12]

Olive leaf extract taken as treatment or to eliminate *in vitro* (in the test tube) colonization is effective against almost all such nosocomial infectious organisms, especially when administered to the most frequent *in vivo* (in the living host) invader, *Staphylococcus aureus.*

Antidoting Staphylococcus Aureus–Caused Colonizations

The bitter glycoside of olive tree products, oleuropein,[13] inhibits the growth of lactic acid bacteria and fungi.[14] Chemically, oleuropein is a molecule that contains glucose, beta-3,4-dihydroxyphenylethyl alcohol, and an acid. Its hydrolysis products include elenolic acid and oleuropein aglycone, which are the active compounds that create antimicrobial responses[15] when applied to *in vitro* growth of *Aspergillus prasiticus*[16] and various strains of lactic acid bacteria.[17] Supported in 1993 by a grant from the European Economic Community, agricultural biochemists C. C. Tassou, Ph.D., and G. J. E. Nychas, Ph.D., published their research report stating without equivocation that the *Staphylococcus aureus* is inhibited in its growth by the phenolics in oleuropein as well as its phenolic extract in broth cultures and in milk. They added, ''The ability of oleuropein to inhibit over a wide pH range gives it the potential to be used in different dairy products as a safeguard against proliferation of *S. aureus.*''[18]

In another 1993 study, conducted at the Division of Biologics, PHLS Centre for Applied Microbiology and Research in Porton Down, Salisbury, Wilts, United Kingdom, it was shown that oleuropein inhibits the growth and enterotoxin B production of *S. aureus.* Even a low concentration of 0.2 percent oleuropein hydrolysis product ''was sufficient to inhibit [*S. aureus*] growth such that the viable [bacterial] count was approximately half that obtained in the control culture without oleuropein while at the same time inhibiting toxin production by a factor of 320,'' wrote the researchers.[19]

Prior to that, a laboratory study demonstrated that there is growth inhibition of *S. aureus* when elenolic acid or aglycone comes in contact with this nosocomial infection producer. By ''inhibition,'' in biochemistry and bacteriology, it's meant that there is a reduction of physiologic activity by either of the hydrolysis product's negative stimulation, causing the stopping or slowing of the rate of spread of the organism.[20]

Two researchers in Perugia, Italy, Federico Federici, Ph.D., and Guido Bongi, Ph.D., had previously identified elenolic acid and oleuropein aglycone as the microorganism-inhibiting hydrolysis products of the olive tree. This information was exceedingly important for the fermentation of Spanish-type green olives. The fermentation rate is influenced by the content of inhibitors of the different olive cultivars, and this knowledge was vital to the olive oil industry.[21]

Olive Leaves' Wash Water Annoys the Olive Oil Industry

As has now become obvious, components of olive leaves effect the olive oil industry. It's been known for at least five decades that something in the olive leaf water used for washing olives, which contains oleuropein, causes the olive oil to become rancid quickly. It turns out that the elenolic acid, aglycone, and other hydrolysis products of oleuropein—which had become part of waste waters of Turkish, American, Greek, Spanish, Portuguese, Albanian, Moroccan, and Italian olive oil mills—adversely affect the biodegradation necessary for oil production. Consequently, such waste waters must be removed or avoided to eliminate any inhibited growth of vegetative cells, as well as the required germination and sporulation processes of organisms for pure olive oil production.[22]

In particular, the multifunctional monoterpene isolated from the several acid-hydrolyzed aqueous extracts of olive leaves, calcium elenolate $[(C^{11}H^{13})^6)^2Ca]$, kills or retards the growth of infectious organisms in humans. The calcium elenolate is the key component that's virucidal, bacteriocidal, fungicidal, and parasiticidal for all those microorganisms against which it has been tested (see Table 10-1 in Chapter 10). It inhibits reverse transcriptases and most other enzymes made by viruses, and it retards the growth of all *Echerichia coli* and *Bacillus subtilis* bacteria strains. As declared by the laboratory scientists at The Upjohn Company, and by biochemists and experimenting clinicians before and after them, this derivative of olive leaf extract has a direct and irreversible adverse effect on the enzymes of those many microorganisms on which it has been tested *in vitro*.[23]

CHAPTER 4

❧

The Olive Leaf Antimicrobials and Those Infectious Diseases They Act Against

In the Southern California town of Fallbrook, agriculturist and herbalist Richard Hall harvests olive leaves for processing into olive leaf extract. "The leaves are harvested only from manzanillo or mission green olive trees as they contain more of the valuable phytochemicals necessary for the most potent extract," says Mr. Hall. "The grove selection plays an important part in assuring that the olive trees are not sprayed with harmful chemicals that might enter a person's body or alter the extract in any way. To assure that no harm comes to the leaves, we only harvest them gently by hand using specially designed gloves."

Other, less careful methods of harvesting produce breakage of the leaves, which begin decaying almost at once and result in loss of medicinal properties. The olive leaves for the American olive leaf concentrate are harvested from 4,500 acres of olive groves located throughout the southern part of California. Because olive leaves resist letting go of their hold on growth and life, some pickers in countries along the Mediterranean sea actually beat the leaves off branches with long sticks.

In Tunisia, the olives and leaves are picked using the

pointed horns of a young goat. The last three inches of the kid's horns are sawed off so that three fingers of the worker's hand may be slipped into the hollow, curved tips. The leaf and olive picker claws the olive tree branches to cause fruit and leaves to fall into waiting baskets below. Such clawing may produce damage to the product's surface which, if present, allows for oxidation along the leaf line. To prevent this damage, any such picking technique is avoided when considering the use of leaves imported from abroad for processing into olive leaf extract.[1]

Inexperienced olive leaf workers are able to pick about twenty pounds in an eight-hour day. Experienced workers usually pick at least twenty-five pounds of leaves per day; the faster the pace of picking, the less expensive will be the final olive leaf extracted product.

"How long olive leaves dry is important for acquiring the most potent extract; therefore, my workers' method of harvesting includes starting the drying process the same day our California leaves are picked, to avoid decay," advises Richard Hall. "I have the leaf pickers use commercial drying in order to control temperatures, thus locking in potency immediately. The American olive leaf product stays freshest that way."

How Olive Leaves Change with Their Environment

Leaves on the olive trees frequently reshape themselves to accommodate changes in their environment. Minute hairs growing around each leaf's pores on its underside are a veritable weather station. During dry periods, the leaf will curl inward to reduce its loss of moisture, and appear its typical olive green in color. When rainfall is abundant, the leaf lays itself open and flat, and the whole tree looks silvery because of the leaves' exposed undersides.

As mentioned in Chapter 2, each olive tree is attacked

by pests, but it does a good job of protecting itself against the varieties that attack its leaves. The key for such protection is that a tree craves sufficient room to grow amid unpolluted air, warm temperatures, bright sunlight, and aerated soil around the roots. A grower of olive trees who provides such ideal conditions will own green riches in the form of abundant fruit, flowing oil from such fruit, and leaves that kill off germs and pests of all types.

If you pass through a grove of olive trees, you might look for the following pests: (1) the bug-eyed olive fly, Dacus, which looks like the common housefly and has three stripes on its chest and sets of lace-patterned wings; (2) the black scale bug, Coccus, which shows an H-shape on her back, making this insect appear as a peppercorn affixed to a twig; (3) a bud-eating moth, the *Prays oleae,* which also likes to eat the olive tree's flowers; (4) appearing like "no seeums" common to the Caribbean islands, the *Liothrips oleae,* are also flying insects too tiny to see, which attempt to foul the olives and curl the leaves; and (5) a small black beetle, the *Phloetribus scarabaeoides,* trying to bore into the wood of the olive tree's branches. Any of these pests are plentiful around trees which lack space, sun, moisture, warmth, and air. Olive trees that grow in ideal conditions have no pests at all or far fewer of them. These are the trees in California from which leaves are harvested for the making of olive leaf extract.[2]

Olive trees are among the world's oldest living species of plant. Some giant trees along the Mediterranean coast, in Europe and North Africa, range from three hundred to eight hundred years old. Most olive tree cultivators agree that the best fruit comes from trees less than eighty years of age, especially if the old wood is pruned away. Such trees produce the finest olive oil.

The olive tree, *Olea europaea* (one of the Oleaceae family of trees), is resistant in nature to insect and microbe attack for another reason that's important to the use of olive leaf extract. Immunity to microbial invasion has been bestowed upon the olive tree because of its high concentration of certain biochemicals, the seco-iridoid glycosides, which occur predominantly in the Oleaceae family. These glycosides are deadly to microorganisms.[3]

The plant's resistance can also be attributed to a large amount of oleanolic acid on and in the foliage, which acts as a barrier to microbial invasion. In the presence of oleanolic acid and its hydrolysis products, microbes cannot germinate and grow. They are inhibited and become dormant or die.[4]

The Onset of Modern Medicinal Uses for Olive Leaves

Knowledge of the medicinal properties of the olive leaf dates back to the early 1800s, as described in the last chapter, when pulverized leaves were used in a green drink to lower high fevers. A couple of decades later, green olive leaves were taken again in liquid form as a treatment for malarial infections. But it wasn't until 1995 that the actual individual therapeutic component in olive leaves—elenolic acid with its salt, calcium elenolate—was uncovered. This discovery now provides the public with a highly effective food supplement which acts as a true illness preventive measure.

It works to stop the onset of such health problems as colds and other viral diseases, fungal, mold, and yeast invasions of many kinds, bacterial infections both minor and major, and protozoan parasitic infestations. Used by itself in a high enough dose, olive leaf extract will expel flukes and other worms invading humans and animals. More than prevention, olive leaf extract offers a new safe and effective therapeutic modality in the ongoing battle against active disease processes.

Below, in Table 1, you are provided with an alphabetical listing of 137 infectious diseases for which olive leaf extract acts effectively as an antimicrobial agent. The listing is taken from numerous published medical sources and from the clinical experiences of currently practicing health professionals who utilize olive leaf extract as part of their armamentarium for patients with internal and external infections, skin diseases, cardiovascular diseases, connective tissue difficulties, and other disorders. Most of all, olive leaf extract is efficacious against infectious diseases, as shown in Table 2.

TABLE 1

Infectious Diseases (Listed Alphabetically) for Which Olive Leaf Extract Acts as an Antimicrobial Agent[5]

- AIDS (Acquired Immunodeficiency Syndrome)
- Amoebiasis
- Anthrax
- Athlete's Foot (Tinea Pedis)
- Bladder Infection (Urinary Tract Infection)
- Botulism
- California Encephalitis (CE)
- Campylobacter (Campylobacteriosis)
- Cat-Scratch Disease
- Chancroid
- Chicken Pox (Varicella)
- Chlamydia
- Chlamydial Pneumonia
- Cholera
- Clostridium Perfringens Infection
- Colds
- Cold Sores (Herpes Simplex I)
- Conjunctivitis (Pink Eye)
- Crabs (Pediculosis Pubis)
- Croup
- Cryptosporidiosis
- Cytomegalovirus (CMV)
- Diarrheal Diseases
- Diphtheria
- Ear Infection (Otitis Media)
- Eastern Equine Encephalitis (EEE)

- Ebola Sudan Virus Infection
- Ebola Zaire Virus Infection
- E. Coli 0157:H7 *(Escherichia coli* Hemorrhagic Colitis 0157:H7
- Encephalitis
- Epstein-Barr Virus (EBV) Infection
- Fifth Disease (Erythema Infectiosum)
- Flu (Influenza)
- Food-Borne Illnesses (Food Poisoning)
- Gastric Ulcers *(Helicobacter pylori)*
- Gastroenteritis (Travelers' Diarrhea)
- Genital Herpes (Herpes Simplex II)
- Genital Warts (Human Papillomavirus, HPV)
- German Measles (Rubella)
- Giardia (Giardiasis)
- Gonorrhea
- Group B Strep Disease
- Hand, Foot, and Mouth Syndrome (Disease)
- Hantavirus Pulmonary Syndrome (HPS)
- Head Lice
- Hepatitis
- Hepatitis A
- Hepatitis B
- Hepatitis C
- Herpes Zoster (Shingles)
- H. Flu Meningitis or Hib (Haemophilus Influenzae Meningitis)
- Impetigo
- Infant Botulism
- Japanese Encephalitis (JE)
- Jock Itch (Tinea Cruris)
- Legionnaires' Disease
- Leprosy (Hansen's Disease)
- Leptospirosis
- Listeria (Listeriosis)
- Lockjaw (Tetanus)
- Lyme Disease
- Lymphocytic Leukemia from Human Acute Leukemia/Lymphoma Virus
- Malaria
- Marburg (Monkey) Virus [*Rhabdovirus simiae*]
- Measles (Rubeola)

- Meningitis, Bacterial
- Meningitis, Viral
- Meningococcal Meningitis
- Mono (Infectious Mononucleosis)
- Mumps
- Mycoplasma Pneumonia
- Newcastle Disease
- Norwalk Agent
- Parrot Fever (Psittacosis)
- Pasteurella (Pasteurellosis)
- PID (Pelvic Inflammatory Disease)
- Pink Eye (Conjunctivitis)
- Pinworm (Enterobiasis)
- Plague
- Pneumococcal Meningitis
- Pneumonia, Broncho, Lobal, or Segmental
- Pneumonia, Bacterial
- Pneumonia, Chlamydial
- Pneumonia, Mycoplasmal
- Pneumonia, Viral
- Polio (Poliomyelitis)
- Pork Tapeworm (Taeniasis)
- Q Fever (Query Fever)
- Rabies
- Rat-Bite Fever
- Rheumatic Fever
- Ringworm (Tinea), of Scalp (Tinea Capitis), of Body (Tinea Corporis)
- Rocky Mountain Spotted Fever
- Roseola (Exanthem Subitem)
- Retrovirus Infection
- Rotavirus Diarrhea
- Roundworm (Toxocariasis)
- RSV (Respiratory Syncytial Virus)
- St. Louis Encephalitis (SLE)
- Salmonella (Salmonellosis)
- Scabies
- Scarlet Fever (Scarlatina)
- Sexually Transmitted Diseases
- Shigella (Shigellosis)
- Shingles (Herpes Zoster)
- Smallpox (Variola)
- Staphylococcal Food Poisoning

- Strep Throat
- Syphilis
- TB (Tuberculosis)
- Thrush (Oral Candidiasis)
- Toxic Shock Syndrome (TSS)
- Toxoplasmosis
- Trich (Trichomoniasis)
- Trichinosis (Trichinellosis)
- Tuberculosis (TB)
- Typhoid Fever
- Urinary Tract Infection (Bladder Infection)
- Vaginal Yeast Infection (Yeast Vaginitis from Candidiasis of the Vagina)
- Vaginitis (Vaginosis)
- Vincent's Infection
- Warts
- Whooping Cough (Pertussis)
- The Yeast Syndrome (Polysystemic Chronic Candidiasis)
- Yellow Fever
- Yersinia (Yersiniosis)

Source: See Chapter 4, reference 5, in the References at the back of the book.

Olive Leaf Extract Cures Diseases Worldwide

Corresponding with me from Budapest, Hungary, Robert Lyons, O.M.D., M.S., Medical Director of The Robert Lyons Clinic, uses acupuncture and herbology for the welfare of his patients. Working with Dr. Lyons are forty wholistic health professionals from the United States. Originally Hungarian-born, these volunteers, both traditionally trained medical doctors and practitioners from other health care professions (chiropractors, naturopaths, homeopaths, nurse practitioners, acupuncturists, podiatrists, dentists, craniologists, herbalists, etc.), have returned to offer improvements in medical services. At the same time, they are enlightening themselves about natural healing agents rather than using synthetic drugs. The Robert Lyons Clinic delivers innovative treatment which is entirely foreign to Central Europe.

Among the medical alternatives the Robert Lyons Clinic employs is the new and potent, but completely safe, antimicrobial agent derived from the olive leaf. As a result of the amazing success experienced throughout Hungary from use of olive leaf extract against all types of infections, the Hungarian government has adopted this over-the-counter herbal food supplement for its Medicare system as the official anti-infectious disease remedy. The cost is so much lower than any prescription drug against infection that the remedy is considered a great boon—a true advancement in health care.

Recently Poland, the Czech Republic, Slovakia, Romania, nearly all of the recently divided countries of Yugoslavia, Russia, Germany, and Italy have begun investigating the efficacy of olive leaf extract.

Case Reports of Hungarian Patients

"My staff and I use many herbal methods of traditional Chinese medicine," said Dr. Robert Lyons, who has a degree in Oriental medicine. "We have carried out a clinical study on five hundred patients using the olive leaf herbal remedy. We dispensed the olive leaf in capsule form and started our patients at a dosage of two capsules three times daily—totaling six capsules per day."

Dr. Lyons reported on his cases from Budapest during my follow-up telephone interview. "Each capsule provides five hundred milligrams of concentrated natural plant extract. When our patients experienced a reduction in their symptoms, we lowered their extract dose to one capsule four times daily.

"The people under treatment responded remarkably well against a variety of microorganisms including many types of viruses, bacteria, yeast, and other fungi. No patients were treated for parasites, but I suspect that olive leaf extract would be effective for those cases of protozoa and helminths, too. The product was incredibly effective against respiratory diseases of bacterial origin, such as tonsilitis, pharangitis, and tracheitis; it improved patients suffering from gastric/duodenal ulcers caused by *Helicobacter pylori;* and it worked just great against viral diseases such as the herpes infections,'' Dr. Lyons said.

"To illustrate my point, let me tell you of one of my patients, a married homemaker, age forty-three, the mother of two teenagers. She had been suffering severely for four years with herpes lesions around her mouth from *Herpes simplex one.* Also, she was terribly uncomfortable from the invasion of *Herpes genitalis* brought home by her husband. And the woman additionally felt great pain from a ring of shingles around her waist caused by *Herpes zoster.* In just seven days,'' continued Dr. Lyons, "the dosage of olive leaf crystalline concentrate that I had administered for her shingles lesions—two capsules thrice daily—cleared up all three herpes infections simultaneously. The lesions for each problem disappeared quickly. This woman reported having no more shingles pain because of the discontinuance of viral blisters. There wasn't any more discomfort around the vagina, and her oral lesions went away. No further signs of herpes of any kind have been apparent in my patient now for over a year.''

Dr. Lyons Is Successful Treating the Yeast Syndrome

"Another patient of mine, a fifty-year-old registered nurse with diabetes mellitus who works in a Budapest hospital, was exhibiting the typical yeast syndrome symptoms produced by *Candida albicans* overgrowth,'' added Dr. Lyons. "Her polysystemic chronic candidiasis had arisen as the result of her long-standing pancreatic dysfunction.

Despite receiving the best of care, the hospital's physicians could do nothing for the woman's generalized yeast condition. Except for local therapy administered to relieve her vaginal itching and discharge, they seemingly failed to recognize that her signs and symptoms came from a systemic fungal disease lodged in the gut.

"The nurse sought help at our Budapest Clinic when her candidiasis finally spread to the mouth as oral thrush," Dr. Lyons explained. "She had heard of our alternative methods of healing. So, spurred by much pain, low-grade fever, night sweats, weakness, and even more difficulties, she consented to follow our clinic's medically innovative route. Having experienced excellent patient responses against the yeast syndrome with applications of olive leaf extract previously, we went directly to that remedy for this nurse.

"What happened? After my patient took the olive leaf extract for four weeks, the yeast syndrome was completely gone from her body. But it didn't end there for me. At a hospital seminar conducted for physicians and nurses, this same young woman stood up and described, with much emotion and many tears of joy, how she was finally rid of the itching, burning, pain, lethargy, and other discomforts of yeast vaginitis and generalized candidiasis," Dr. Lyons confirmed. "I was sitting in the audience. When my health professional peers turned to look at me as some kind of medical hero, I had an incredible feeling of pride. They wanted to know how I managed the successful treatment. So I told them about olive leaf extract for curing the yeast syndrome."

This doctor of Oriental medicine went on to chart the progress of his administration of olive leaf extract to all five hundred clinical patients in his single-blind study. The Hungarians, suffering a variety of diseases, not knowing what remedy they were being dispensed, followed directions and took the gray/green-colored gelatin capsules as if they were vitamins. Dr. Robert Lyon was highly gratified by the remedy's therapeutic effects. Table 2 shows results he

TABLE 2

Results from the Use of Olive Leaf Extract Against Pathological Organisms—Viruses, Bacteria, and Fungi

Disease Entities	No. of Patients	Fully Recovered	Improved	Unchanged	Deteriorated
Respiratory diseases (tonsilitis, pharyngitis, tracheitis, etc.)	119	115	4	none	none
Lung conditions (pneumonia, bronchitis, etc.)	45	42	3	none	none
Dental problems (pulpitis, leukoplakia, stomatitis)	67	60	5	2	none
Skin conditions (herpes and other viral skin problems)	172	120	52	none	none
Bacterial skin infections (pyoderma, injuries)	37	30	7	none	none
Ulcer disease (while experiencing *Helicobacter pylori* infection)	17	none	17	none	none
Strengthened immunity	43	N.A.	40	3	none

From the above results, the Clinic's conclusions are:

1. The rate of improvement and recovery from all bacterial and viral infections was approximately 98 percent.
2. For all patients involved in this clinical study, the body's immune system was strengthened.
3. Including children and adolescents among the tested patients, none experienced any adverse side effects.

Characteristics of the study's patients—

Gender:	58% women,	42% men
Ages:	10 to 20 years:	12
	20 to 30 years:	117
	30 to 40 years:	143
	40 to 50 years:	181
	50 and over:	47
	Number of patients:	500

Source: A Clinical Investigation by the Robert Lyons Clinic of Budapest, Hungary—Robert Lyons, O.M.D., M.S., was the chief investigator.

experienced from use of olive leaf extract, which he and his colleagues consider a highly satisfying clinical study.

As you'll learn in chapters to follow, such excellent results as described by Dr. Robert Lyons and presented in Table 2 are common for the therapeutic administration of olive leaf extract against viral infections, bacterial infections, yeast syndrome, and other diseases.

Olive leaf extract, this natural crystalline concentrate, has undergone much investigation, and has been produced as bulk powder, liquid, tablets, tincture, tea, nasal spray, and more. After 142 years of experimentation, it's been prepared as a gelatin capsule for oral administration. The product is being considered for dispensing to patients attending private clinics and hospitals throughout nearly all the Baltic States. The Hungarian government has made olive leaf extract a standard treatment for infections in its national health insurance program. In addition, other countries are considering adopting the product as their official antimicrobial medicare remedy.

Until now, just a few health professionals in the wholistic medical community in North America have been aware of the benefits accruing from the use of olive leaf extract. This book should go a long way toward educating many more of them.

At the opening of this chapter I described the many intricate steps in the olive leaf's harvesting and processing so as to keep its potency intact. The final, pure, encapsulated olive leaf product was finally approved for packaging and worldwide wholesale distribution during the spring of 1995. Because there had been so little information made available to medical consumers until now, it was only beginning to be distributed through health food stores in North America and on other continents during the summer of 1996. This book may be bringing vital information to the attention of people everywhere for their improved health and welfare. As a result, olive leaf extract is fast becoming the most exciting product distributed by the health food industry worldwide.

CHAPTER 5

❧

Additional Therapeutic Applications for the Olive Leaf Concentrate

During an interview from his home in Malibu, California, retired postal inspector Morris Corrs, age seventy-two, described his bout with a series of health problems. He had been forced to take early retirement from the United States postal system twelve years before because of the double atherosclerotic difficulties, coronary heart disease (CHD), and peripheral vascular disease (PVD). For these two serious illnesses, he had undergone individual surgical operations: coronary artery bypass of three blood vessels to the heart and femoral artery bypasses in the left and right thighs. In all instances, the operations had been only marginally helpful. He still experienced periodic angina pectoris in the chest and intermittent claudication of both limbs.

Angina pectoris is a cramping pain in the chest caused most often by a shortage of oxygen to the heart (myocardial anoxia). It is often linked with hardening of the arteries (atherosclerosis) of the heart and the pain usually travels down the inside of the left arm. It often occurs with a feeling of suffocation and impending death. Attacks of angina pectoris are related to exertion, emotional stress, and contact with intense cold.

Intermittent claudication is pain of the legs with cramps in the calves caused by poor circulation of the blood (also from atherosclerosis). The pain alternates between periods of activity and inactivity associated with walking, and may include lameness or limping. It is relieved by rest, but confines the victim to only limited use of his lower limbs.

Mr. Corrs suffered not only from CHD and PVD but also had chronic joint pain in both knees and various discomforting lower leg nerve sensations (parasthesias). His desire was to advise me about how all four conditions improved from his steadily taking capsules of olive leaf extract on a regular basis, which he is continuing to do.

"Upon the recommendation of Isaac David Freez, N.D., my Southern California naturopath, I took olive leaf extract just to see what would happen to my chest pain and intermittent claudication," Mr. Corrs said. "I never popped down more than one capsule per day until recently, when I decided to increase my dosage to two a day as an assist for my aching knees. I was experiencing prolonged knee discomfort from an accident I had sustained six months before. As a result of the knee injury, I was feeling sensations of pins and needles in my legs, feet, and toes. In addition to having the joint pain and nerve pain in both legs, I was undergoing intermittent claudication as a result of my clogged arteries from peripheral vascular disease. Occasionally angina chest pain struck me too.

"Now, however, from taking the olive leaf extract, all four of my health problems are either diminished or have disappeared altogether. My chest pains and leg cramps are so much better. I've not had angina pain for four months when there was a time I felt it several times a week and had to put nitroglycerine under my tongue. I've not needed nitro for all of these months. As for my legs, today I'm able to walk a full mile without stopping to recover, when previously it was difficult for me to go more than a city block. If I tried, I'd feel calf pain from intermittent claudication," assured Morris Corrs. "The knee pain went away after only two weeks of doubling my dose of the extract and, subsequently, the pins and needles sensation has gone too.

"I now stock capsules of olive leaf extract and give them to anyone requiring help for heart trouble, leg cramps, arthritis, bursitis, other chronic joint pains, infections of all types, boosting energy, and much more. Once the news gets out about olive leaf extract, I'm sure that this product will be declared the finest health discovery made in the twenty-first century," affirms Morris Corrs.

The Coronary Dilating Action of Olive Leaf Extract

Laboratory experiments were conducted in Sofia, Bulgaria, at the Institute of Physiology, Bulgarian Academy of Sciences, during 1977, to determine the pharmacological actions of certain plant substances for their coronary dilating and antiarrhythmic effects. The investigations were carried out on the hearts of laboratory rabbits bred for that purpose. Used in the studies were materials coming from valerian roots *(Valeriana officinalis),* all the crataemon and hyperoside flavonoids obtained from hawthorn berries *(Crataegus monogina),* and iridoid oleuropein isolated from olive leaves *(Olea europaea).* The experimenters determined that oleuropein produces a clear-cut coronary dilatatory action.

When oleuropein is administered to the hearts of rabbits, their coronary artery blood flow increases by more than 50 percent. The same effect takes place in cats. Oleuropein was active against barium chloride–induced arrhythmia (in rabbits) and against calcium-induced arrhythmia (in rats). Oleuropein produced a pronounced and long-lasting effect of lowering elevated blood pressure in wakeful dogs.[1]

The investigators reported that oleuropein is exceedingly safe since its intraperitoneal (i.p.) injection dosage offers an LD^{50} for mice of 2,000 mg/kg as compared to hawthorn, which is less safe, with an i.p. LD^{50} of 1,650 mg/kg and safer still than valerian root, with its i.p. LD^{50} of 450 mg/kg. With oral administration of the three plant substances to mice, the olive leaf's oleuropein level of safety is an astoundingly high 4,000 mg/kg.[2] This level of safety makes olive leaf extract safer to take orally than drinking tap water in New York City (which is proud of its tap water purity).

Olive Leaf Components Lower High Blood Pressure

The health professional in whom Morris Corrs has a great deal of confidence, Dr. Isaac David Freez, naturopath and colon hydrotherapist of Santa Barbara, California, stated, "I don't oversell olive leaf extract but simply present it as an option for a variety of health problems. Certainly it's useful for colds, flu, and other infections, including traveler's diarrhea. I do find olive leaf extract lowers hypertension, so my patients with high blood pressure are told to take it as an adjunctive remedy for their difficulty, along with eating the Mediterranean diet."

The effect of olive leaf extract on hypertension has been tested extensively in laboratory animals. High blood pressure induced in adult Wistar rats comes down when a decoction of olive leaves is administered. The *decoction* consisted of boiling and straining olive leaves and mixing them in a proportion of 50 grams to 1000 milliliters (ml) of water. This hypotensive finding for olive leaves was proven in experiments carried out during July 1990 at the Department of Pharmacology, School of Pharmacy, University of Granada, in Spain. The experimenters also showed that oleuropeoside, another component present in olive leaf extract, is responsible for a vasodilator effect on the smooth muscle layer (the endothelium) of animal arteries. Oleuropeoside pulls down elevated blood pressure by causing constricted arteries to become more flexible and relax.[3]

In prior laboratory studies conducted at the Department

of Experimental and Clinical Pharmacology of the Postgraduate Medical Institute in Sofia, Bulgaria, it was learned that oleuropein reduces elevated blood pressure by an average of 68 percent of the initial hypertensive level in fully conscious dogs.

At the same institution, anesthetized hypertensive rats injected with a dose of 30 mg/kg of oleuropein displayed a gradual fall of blood pressure by 33 percent. Then, experiments with hypertensive anesthetized cats using the same dosage of olive leaf extract as in the rats provoked a slow but steady fall of blood pressure by 36 percent of the initial level.[4]

The Bulgarian investigators, Victor Petkov, Ph.D., D.Sc., and Peter Manolov, Ph.D., also reported the animals' coronary blood flow improved from the use of their oleuropein injections, especially in rabbits. They exhibited antiarrhythmic action as well, wherein an irregular heart beat corrected itself.[5]

After his first ground-breaking publication, Dr. Petkov went on to investigate fifty plants growing in Bulgaria and in other countries which furnish hypotensive, anti-atheromatous, and coronary artery–dilating actions. His enthusiasm for olive leaves, published in the 1979 issue of the *American Journal of Chinese Medicine,* has never been picked up and acted upon by American scientists. That's a shame, because almost twenty years have been lost in which millions of people throughout the world could have had their elevated blood pressures lowered to normal, their atherosclerotic arteries unhardened, and their heart arteries dilated without resorting to life-threatening coronary artery bypass surgery.

Dr. Petkov writes: "Olive leaves, *Folia oleae,* applied in the form of decoction or tincture are recommended as an antihypertensive remedy. This healing effect of olive leaves was described as far back as 1935 by the French phytotherapeutist Leclerc. It was thought that the hypotensive effect is due to the choline-like substances contained in the olive leaves." Dr. Petkov went on to advise that the iridoid oleuropein isolated from olive leaves is a promising natural substance for bringing high blood pressure to normal, causing a dilating effect in constricted arteries, and straightening out irregular heartbeats as in arrhythmias causing atrial fibrillation.[6]

The olive leaf's ability to lower pathological levels of blood pressure has been known since 1951,[7] although oleuropein as the particular hypotensive ingredient was not recognized until nine years later.[8] Now this advantageous medical action of olive leaf extract is well established.

Olive Leaf Ingredients Eliminate Atrial Fibrillation

Sixty-one-year-old Collin Hargraves, a shoe clerk trying to continue working in Saskatoon, Saskatchewan, Canada, has been the victim of atrial fibrillation for two years and nothing in the allopathic medical armamentarium helped him. "The medical profession has given up on me completely. I've taken all of the available prescribed drugs: digoxin, beta blockers, the calcium antagonists, anticoagulants, and more. When I refused the implantation of a permanent pacemaker, two top cardiologists from this region said they couldn't do anything for me and advised that I get my family and financial affairs in order," Mr. Hargraves explained. "They told my wife and me that there is no hope for correcting the atrial fibrillation."

Atrial fibrillation is a heart condition marked by rapid, unsystematic contractions of the upper heart chambers (the atria). This causes the lower chambers (the ventricles) to beat irregularly, at a rate of 130 to 150 beats per minute. The atria may discharge more than 350 electric impulses a minute. The lower chambers cannot contract in response to all these impulses and the contractions become disordered. The rapid pulsations result in a decreased amount of blood pumped to the body. The disorganized contractions of the atria can cause blood clots to form in the atria and bring about extremely serious heart disorders, such as mitral stenosis and/or atrial infarction, both of which are life-threatening.[9]

"Based on the cardiologists' verdicts, I've sought out health care from a specialist in alternative medicine. Olive leaf extract was my wholistic physician's recommendation, and it's worked well for my atrial fibrillation," states Mr. Hargraves. "After taking olive leaf extract capsules for three months, I can chop wood, take long walks, and do chores around the house, when none of those activities could I do before. The heart palpitations, weakness, faintness, and shortness of breath always stopped me then. Those symptoms have gone away. My physician read your two articles, Dr. Walker, the first in the *Townsend Letter for Doctors & Patients*[10] and the second in *Explore! for the Professional.*[11] Recognizing from those journal articles that arrhythmia— my personal health problem—responds to olive leaf extract, the physician suggested this product, and it's a good thing for me that she did.

Oleuropein Stops LDL Cholesterol from Oxidizing

By now you know that the bitter principle of olives, oleuropein, is a major component of the polyphenolic fraction of olive oil and an extract of the olive leaf. The chemically processed natural substance, labeled by biochemists in the olive oil industry as *oleuropein*$^{10-5}$M, effectively inhibits a biochemical response produced in the laboratory, the copper sulphate–induced, low-density lipoprotein (LDL) oxidation reaction. A published study conducted at the University of Milan in the Institute of Pharmacological Sciences indicates that oleuropein interferes with biochemical events that are implicated in hardening of the arteries (atherogenic disease). There is a direct therapeutic connection between the use of olive leaf extract and the prevention of peripheral vascular disease and coronary artery disease affecting the heart.[12]

Another study's authors, Valentina Ruiz-Gutierrez, Ph.D., Francisco J. G. Muriana, Ph.D., Roberto Maestro, Ph.D., and Enrique Graciani, Ph.D., confirm that, "Pre-incubation of LDL with oleuropein, at concentrations as low as 10^{-5}M, significantly retarded vitamin E loss and associated lipid peroxidation."[13]

The Antioxidant Effect of Oleuropein

When it comes to an antioxidant effect, oleuropein acts in a fashion similar to that of various flavonoids.[14] Metal ion chelation therapy created by olive leaf extract makes an important contribution to reversing atherosclerosis, but other processes, such as chain-breaking of free radical propagation, also work against hardening of the arteries.[15]

There is a goodly quantity of phenols (chemical components making up flavonoids) in products coming from the olive tree. Nutritional scientists' published observations that intakes of a few milligrams per day of flavonoids in other substances is correlated with a lower incidence of peripheral vascular disease and coronary heart disease indicates that the daily intake of olive oil and/or olive leaf extract containing phenols will likely bring on a similar result.[16]

Finally, as mentioned previously, waste water from washing olives after picking and before pressing for oil is a major problem in the olive oil industry. Any of the waste water coming in contact with olives prior to their pressing effectively stops the desirable fermentation of olive oil. The washing procedure is called *malaxation*. Malaxation gives rise to a waste-water extract that's loaded not only with antimicrobials but also with natural antioxidants. There was further testing of the waste waters by University of Milan investigators with a model of lipid peroxidation. In their experiments they caused copper sulphate–induced oxidation of the lipids, which when mixed with olive leaf extract, gave rise to powerful antioxidant activity.[17]

The olive leaf extract derived from crystallizing the malaxation waste provides a cheap but powerful, as yet unused, source of natural antioxidants. The olive compound acts as a free radical scavenger, or as a metal ion oral chelator, thus inhibiting the superoxide-driven reactions. The waste-water components derived from washing olives function as chain-breaking agents, in a fashion similar to that proposed as the biochemical physiological action of the alpha, beta, gamma, and other tocopherols in vitamin E.[18]

Olive Leaf Application for Peptic Ulcer and Hiatal Hernia

Residing in Sacramento, California, seventy-year-old Frank Chisholm, a politician often visiting the state capitol building, was suffering from symptoms of two gastrointestinal disorders, peptic ulcer and hiatal hernia. During the six years that Mr. Chisholm has felt these gut discomforts of chronic indigestion with heartburn, he underwent surgery for each of them. The two operations didn't solve anything.

Peptic ulcer, a break in the mucous lining of the alimentary tract, fails to heal and is often accompanied by inflammation. There's an ongoing digestion of the mucosa by the enzyme pepsin and acid, which are present in unusually high concentrations. For Mr. Chisholm, peptic acid was present in his esophagus (gullet) as an esophageal ulcer, associated with gastroesophageal reflux or *reflux esophagitis* (both reflux types causing awful heartburn) from his hiatal hernia.

Hiatal hernia is the passage of a part of the stomach through the hole (hiatus) for the esophagus. Often the only treatment other than surgery is chiropractic manipulation to push back the intruding stomach portion from the esophagus. However, the adjustment holds for only a short time, perhaps one week.

"A year and a half ago I began to once again experience excrutiating pain when I ate. One bite of toast in the morning would leave me uncomfortable for the rest of the day," said Mr. Chisholm. "It's true that I function in a stressful atmosphere at my occupation. I've tried every antacid that the pharmaceutical companies invent, but they don't do the job for me. Yet, my suffering stopped after my wife recommended that I take this grayish-green powder in a gelatin capsule, olive leaf extract. In five minutes my abdominal pain was gone. And the comfort lasted for much of the morning, at which time I took another capsule.

"The next day I took the olive leaf extract before breakfast, and I had no problems during or after any of my meals. The burning pain does not come anymore if I'm faithful about taking the olive leaf extract as a prophylactic measure against heartburn," affirms Frank Chisholm.

Olive Leaf Extract Is Specific For Eliminating Psoriasis

A dermatologist in Elmwood Park, New Jersey, Joseph J. Territo, M.D., states: "I have used the olive leaf extract, *Olea europeae*, for better than one hundred patients. My primary goal was to observe its effectiveness on psoriasis, because olive leaf extract incorporated into a gel acts as an anti-inflammatory agent, but both the tablets and capsules are effective.

"My experience in using olive leaf extract capsules indicates that patients exhibit an improvement in their psoriasis of up to 70 percent. I've witnessed improvement not only in the reduction of psoriatic scales but also in the skin's erythema [redness] related to them, and also in a lessening of the inflammatory response. With the olive leaf capsules taken internally and the olive leaf gel applied topically, my patients have an even greater improvement in their psoriasis lesions—as much as a 75 percent success ratio," Dr. Territo reports. "I believe the excellent results are holding for my patients, and I've been dispensing the olive leaf ingredients for over a year-and-a-half now. I was perhaps the first physician in the United States to test olive leaf extract.

"Added to the fine results of applying olive leaf extract for psoriasis, I also have excellent patient responses to its usage for the treatment of fibromyalgia," additionally suggests Dr. Joseph Territo. "I'm anxious to spread the word about the therapeutic benefits of olive leaf extract."

Olive Leaf Extract Relieves Fibromyalgia

Writing from Akron, Ohio, Robert Fallaci, a plumber, age forty-two, states: "I became ill with stomach and prostate infections in December of 1993, which were treated by my medical doctor with high doses of antibiotics. The infectious symptoms never seemed to completely go away, however, and then more discomforts struck in different parts of my body. I came down with chronic back and neck pain, flu-like symptoms, swollen glands, sinusitis, digestive difficulties, including diarrhea and heartburn. Most of all I felt tender points, tightness, and spasms in the muscles. I was subsequently diagnosed at the Cleveland Clinic a year-and-a-half later as having been hit by a collective series of illness—a syndrome—which the doctors on the clinic's staff called 'fibromyalgia.'"

Fibromyalgia is actually myofascial pain syndrome, or fibromyositis, a group of common nonarticular rheumatic disorders characterized by achy pain, tenderness, and stiffness of the muscles, in the areas of tendon insertions, and in adjacent soft-tissue structures. These painful sensations may be the primary generalized problem or be concomitant with another associated or underlying conditions. The discomfort could also be localized, and often related to overuse or microtrauma factors.

To be most accurate, fibromyalgia indicates pain in

fibrous tissues, muscles, tendons, ligaments, and other "white" connective tissues. Various combinations of these conditions may occur together as muscular rheumatism, and any of the fibromuscular tissues may be involved, but those in the low back (lumbago), neck (neck pain or spasm), shoulders, thorax, and thighs (charley horses) are especially affected. A viral or systemic infection such as Lyme disease often brings on fibromyalgia.

"Physicians at the Cleveland Clinic prescribed a diverse set of drugs for me, such as Prozac-type antidepressants, anti-inflammatory agents, among which were corticosteroids, and other toxic agents. I refused to take any of them," writes Mr. Fallaci. "I began taking olive leaf extract along with my regular vitamin and mineral supplements on August 20, 1995, at the rate of one tablet every six hours. I increased the dosage after five days and began feeling better. The achiness lessened. I tried different dosages for a week until I found the optimum amount for me. Today I take three capsules four times a day (total of twelve daily) and stay on olive leaf extract as maintenance.

"My overall health has greatly improved, and now I feel wonderful. Muscle spasms and tenderness don't trouble me anymore. The olive leaf extract has given me lots of energy, and improved my disposition too, because pain is never a factor for me," Robert Fallaci says.

"Something else—my fingernails had been riddled with fungus infection for ten years, leaving them wrinkled, discolored, flaking detritus, and awful looking. From using olive leaf extract to cure my fibromyalgia, my fingernails have grown out absolutely normal looking. They've returned to a normal shape and color," the man added. "My fingernail fungus is cured."

The Recommended Dosage of Olive Leaf Extract

I personally take olive leaf extract daily, in a maintenance program against getting infections of any kind. Each day under usual conditions of stress, my dosage is two capsules. I ingest one capsule on an empty stomach upon arising, (about 7:00 A.M.) and a second capsule approximately two-and-a-half hours after lunch (about 3:30 P.M.). If I'm traveling overseas or around the United States on an assignment, or if I commute into New York City to consult with one of my publishers, I increase my dosage by at least half (three capsules daily). In my experience, olive leaf extract furnishes extra energy to sustain me against the stress of travel, and to cope with the vast amount of pollutants and germs present in any major metropolitan area.

The Southern California physician James R. Privitera, M.D., who utilizes olive leaf extract for his patients, and markets a brand of the product under his personal label, has this to say about dosage:

Olive leaf extract is currently available in the form of 500 mg. tablets. The routine dosage is one tablet every six hours, or four throughout the day. Take the supplement between meals for best results. In the case of bad colds or flu, you can use two tablets every six hours. For acute infections, some individuals have taken more—three and even four every six hours—and reported rapid relief. If you encounter a ''die-off'' effect, cut back on the number of tablets you are taking, or temporarily discontinue them. For healthy folks seeking more energy or the preventive benefits of olive leaf extract, we suggest one or two tablets a day. The younger and cleaner the body, the more responsive it is to supplements such as this. When a person becomes older and more toxic, more of the supplement is required to do the job.[19]

A medical facility which dedicates itself largely to wholistic health care practices, the Nevada Clinic in Las Vegas, Nevada, utilizes olive leaf extract for many of its patients, in particular those suffering from infections of all types. The administrator of the Nevada Clinic furnishes a written recommendation of dosages to the clinic's patients. Here is the information that the clinic's administrator hands out for the treatment of an illness:

> *Recommended dosing is four 500 mg capsules throughout the day or one every six hours. It [olive leaf extract] is best taken before or between meals. For acute flu symptoms, take two capsules every six hours. For acute [bacterial or viral] infections, more rapid relief may be obtained by taking three or more capsules every six hours. Healthy individuals need only take one or two capsules a day to benefit from the supplement's energizing and/or preventive effect. In general, the older and more toxic the individual, the more resistance present in the body and hence, the more of the supplement that will be required for optimal results. In the event of a "die-off" effect (a natural detoxification response by the body) generated by the olive leaf supplement, the number of capsules taken should be reduced or temporarily discontinued.*

Table 3 offers you an insight into the exact components in the nutritional supplement formulation of olive leaf extract made into tablets. More makers of olive leaf extract are entering the field monthly as the product grows in popularity.

TABLE 3

Components Often Present in Tablets of Olive Leaf Extract

The following formula of nutritional components and excipients may be present in olive leaf extract tablets:

Olive Leaf Granulation	505 mg
Cellulose	50 mg
Stearic Acid (vegetable)	13 mg
Croscarmellose sodium	13 mg
Silicon dioxide	8 mg
Magnesium stearate (vegetable)	7 mg
Maltodextrin 10 DE	4 mg
Total core weight	600 mg

Oleuropein Concentrations in Olive Leaf Extract

It is apparent that there are numerous active and synergistic components at work in olive leaf extract. When it comes to identifying a high-quality olive leaf extract product, these active ingredients can be very helpful. That's because some constituents, while not solely responsible for all of olive leaf's medicinal effects, are excellent indicators of overall activity.

As stated elsewhere in this book, studies have shown that oleuropein has significant therapeutic activity against bacterial, fungal, protozoan, and viral infections. An extract product with a good concentration of oleuropein therefore should be quite effective; however, more is not always better. An increase in the concentration of one component in olive leaf extract is unavoidably at the expense of other important components. Thus, it would be far less desirable to use an extract with a concentration of 99 percent oleuropein, because such an extract would have 1 percent or less of all other synergistic ingredients needed for optimal activity.

Currently, throughout the United States, there are many forms of olive leaf extract being sold in pharmacies and health food stores. One indicator of high quality olive leaf extract is the concentration of oleuropein. While other oleuropein concentrations can be high quality, a 6 percent concentration has been found effective.

Such moderate levels of oleuropein are stable, cost effective, and denote a strong concentration of active principles. This level of oleuropein also indicates that other synergistic cofactors have most likely not been sacrificed. Also, as indication of high quality olive leaf extract is the manufacturer. A conscientious manufacturer with a history of selling excellent products will likely produce a high quality of olive leaf extract.

PART TWO

Successful Antimicrobial Therapy for Viral, Bacterial, Fungal, and Parasitic Illnesses

CHAPTER 6

✌

You Can Stop Herpes and Other Viral Diseases from Threatening Your Loved Ones

In San Mateo, California, Bernard Friedlander, A.P.T., D.C., practices a highly sophisticated form of chiropractic medicine that includes recent advances in nutritional healing. He includes sports nutrition, molecular biology, and the most current discoveries of healthful phytochemicals as part of his therapeutic programs.

During the summer of 1995, thirty-four-year-old Vivian Platt, the vice-president of product design for a Silicon Valley computer company, returned to Dr. Friedlander sooner than her regularly scheduled appointments required. As a means of keeping fit, she had been taking prophylactic chiropractic spinal adjustments from him every two weeks. This time the woman was afraid she had contracted a sexually transmitted disease.

For the prior two months, Ms. Platt had been engaged in a torrid sexual relationship. This had continued until her partner broke out in the telltale blisters of genital herpes. Only when she spotted them did she learn she was being intimately exposed to this communicable disease. That same day, she consulted Dr. Friedlander for whatever preventive treatment was available.

The Symptom Complex of Herpes Genitalis

As an infection caused by the herpes simplex virus type 2 (HSV-II), *herpes genitalis* almost invariably gets passed along by sexual contact. It is moderately contagious and produces painful blisters on the skin and moist lining of the sex organs. Herpes genitalis is usually transmitted by sexual contact between a man and woman, and symptoms appear within four to seven days after exposure. The condition tends to recur because this virus establishes a latent infection of the sacral sensory nerve ganglia, from which it reactivates and reinfects the skin. Thus, it lives inside the nerve cells, where the attack cells of the immune system cannot find it.

When acquired during pregnancy, HSV-II may transmigrate from the mother's blood to the fetus or to the newborn by direct contact with the mother's infected tissue (along the birth canal) during birth. The new baby will have congenital herpes of the genitalia.

In the man, herpes genitalis infections usually resemble penile ulcers. A small group of blisters surrounded by redness of the skin often occurs on the tip or foreskin of the penis. These turn into surface sores that will heal in five to seven days, although they also may become infected. The sores are painful and are sometimes accompanied by a burning sensation, urinary problems, fever, illness, and swelling of the lymph nodes in the groin area.

The female patient frequently has symptoms the same as, or similar to, the male. Members of both sexes will usually complain to attending physicians of painful sexual intercourse. In a woman, herpes genitalis lesions are likely to appear as groups of scabbed or open sores on the surfaces of the cervix, vagina, or perineum. There will sometimes be a discharge from the cervix, and vaginal blisters may appear as mucous open sores. For both sexes, this particular herpes simplex virus tends to cause repeated attacks at regular intervals—monthly, bimonthly, or trimonthly.[1]

Recognizing her own exposure, Vivian Platt did not wait to experience any outbreak of herpes genitalis. She consulted Dr. Bern Friedlander right away. Standard medical treatment of genital herpes sores is with the antibiotic acyclovir, administered in intravenous, oral, or topical form. Being a chiropractor, Dr. Friedlander resorted to another, more effective, safer, and relatively inexpensive preventive remedy. It's a nutritional supplement offering no adverse side effects, which he had used before with remarkable success for other viral, bacterial, fungal, candidial, and protozoan infections. Indeed, this heretofore unrecognized product exhibits multitudinous antimicrobial attributes *par excellence.*

The result was that Ms. Platt never suffered any signs or symptoms of genital herpes. The sexually transmitted disease was prevented from developing as a result of her taking the compound made from olive leaves. "Nearly twenty months have passed, and no herpes genitalis lesions have made themselves known," said Dr. Friedlander. "Although there was strong potential for the condition to make an appearance, my patient never went through any herpes infection. The simplest nutraceutical substance one could imagine—an extract of the olive leaf—preserved the patient's health.

"I've seen this happen frequently with my use of olive leaf extract. Its effect is subtle but amazing," Dr. Friedlander concluded. "The compound has been useful for eliminating the symptoms of all types of infections including yeast, fungal, bacterial, viral, and parasitic, plus chronic fatigue syndrome, rheumatoid arthritis, prostate cancer, some other cancers, skin eruptions, psoriasis, fibromyositis, and more. In my chiropractic practice, I've grown to depend on this extract of olive leaves, especially for health problems arising from most types of viral attacks—even for the common cold."

The prevention or treatment of sexually transmitted diseases (STDs) by the use of olive leaf extract seems to be an advantageous application of this natural substance. And its use is not limited to genital herpes. Below, Table 4 lists the STDs responsive to olive leaf extract by genital disease category.

During the past twenty years, STDs have evolved from the classic venereal diseases of gonorrhea, syphilis, chancroid, lymphogranuloma venereum, and granuloma inguinale, to a much broader group of illnesses. The newer definition of SDTs encompasses virtually all pathogens that may be transmitted through human-to-human contact during intimate sexual activity, including those illnesses produced by bacteria, fungi, ectoparasites, protozoans, and viruses. All of them respond in some measure to the oral ingeston of olive leaf extract. If for no other reason, olive leaf extract should be taken to lessen the symptoms of infection.

Sexually transmitted diseases are contagious and usually caught by sexual intercourse or other genital contact. These infections derived from various microbes, and previously referred to as venereal diseases, are quite common, as you'll learn in chapters farther along.

Heterosexual transmission of the human immunodeficiency virus (HIV) infection has been thought of by authorities as an SDT. It's especially tragic when passed along to the fetus during pregnancy. This has become a major obstetric problem, because it occurs in nearly half of the children born to HIV+ mothers, resulting in an aggressive, shortened disease course in the child that usually ends in death before the age of two years. Because of the high risk of fetal transmission, termination of pregnancy is generally advocated by obstetricians once the diagnosis is confirmed.

How Viruses Are Different from Any Other Life Form

Viruses are unique organisms in that they are near the center of the entire process that comprises life. Unlike worms, protozoa, bacteria, or yeasts, molds, and other

TABLE 4

Sexually Transmitted Diseases (STDs) Which May Respond to Olive Leaf Extract as Prevention/Treatment

Illnesses Are Listed According to the Primary Lesion or Tissue Location of the Disease Symptoms

ULCERATIVE GENITAL DISEASES
    Syphilis
      Syphilis and HIV
    Chancroid
    Granuloma Inguinale
    Genital Herpes
      Herpes and HIV

GENITAL MUCOSAL DISEASES
    Gonorrhea
    Chlamydia
    Mycoplasmas

EPIDERMAL DISEASES
    Human Papillomavirus
    Molluscum Contagiosum
    Ectoparasitic Diseases
      Lice
      Scabies

ENTERITIS/DIARRHEAL SYNDROMES

VAGINAL DISEASES
    Vulvovaginal Candidiasis
    Trichomoniasis
    Bacterial Vaginosis

Millions of people infected with STDs are asymptomatic for long periods of time and go undiagnosed but continue to transmit the infecting agent. Multiple infections may occur simultaneously. *Chlamydia trachomatis* is the most common STD in the United States and many other Western industrialized nations._____

Source: F. J. Palella and R. L. Murphy, "Sexually transmitted diseases." In *The Biologic and Clinical Basis of Infectious Diseases,* 5th edition. Editors S. T. Shulman, J. P. Phair, L. R. Peterson, and J. R. Warren (Philadelphia: W. B. Saunders Co., 1997), p. 208; M. Walker. "Olive leaf extract: The new oral treatment to counteract most types of pathological organisms." *Explore! for the Professional* 7(4):31–37, Oct. 1996.

fungi—which invade an animal's body tissues; are attached by the host's immune mechanism, and are then cleared from the body as waste products—viruses often enter and remain in the body's cells. As long as they are part of a human host—in the blood, cells, lymph, bone marrow, or any other functioning tissue—viruses threaten that person's state of health.

Getting rid of symptoms related to the viral infection doesn't mean that the virus is eliminated. The virus can remain dormant and break out again when the host's immunity becomes compromised. Once a viral disease has invaded, the individual's homeostasis and prolonged wellness remain in danger of breaking down once again with signs and symptoms of disease.[2]

A virus is the simplest form of life—a piece of genetic material surrounded by a small protein "envelope" or coat. Unlike the nine other microorganisms described in Chapter 1, viruses go directly inside the body's cellular structures. They cannot multiply outside of a living body. Outside the host, viruses can exist only in the form of minute invisible crystals. In this dry crystalline form, viruses don't multiply. But once they return to a living host, the viruses can activate, enter the host cells, subdivide, and produce pathology. For example, herpes zoster (shingles) is believed to come from reactivation of the varicella (chicken pox) virus lying dormant in cells of a dorsal root ganglion (a section of nerve).[3] Chicken pox can occur at any age, but it's most common in children from two to eight years old. Therefore, shingles in adults may result from the herpes virus waiting to strike from childhood onward.[4]

If left alone and not endangered by an adverse environment, viruses are almost immortal. Recently, some Italian investigators discovered intact smallpox viruses in a human mummy from about 1000 A.D. The scientists were astonished to discover that they were able to culture the viral crystals and infect living cells with them.

Stopping HIV and Other Viral Impregnations of Genes

In the United States, researchers have taken chromosomes from the brain cells of preserved ancient Indians found in a Florida grave; they successfully cloned these genes in the laboratory. The gene core of viruses is a nonliving piece of information. When it gets into a body, it enters the nucleus of cells and becomes part of the person's own genes.

To illustrate this point, realize that once the human immunodeficiency virus (HIV) gets inside someone, it will probably be there for the rest of that person's life. This circumstance remains in effect unless something gets absorbed into his or her cells that kills the HIV (see Chapter 8). There's a certain chemical ingredient in the leaves of olive trees—the salt of a leaf's chemically reacted hydrolysis product, elenolic acid—that I've referred to as *calcium elenolate*. When released, calcium elenolate does just what's required against the virus; it's virucidal. If calcium elenolate has been absorbed into your tissues, the offending virus can't invade cells because it's killed by the presence of this virucidal substance.

If there isn't any virucidal substance available, HIV will possibly penetrate the cellular structure. Then, often it gets passed on to the offspring of an infected person. (New York City alone is currently attempting to cope with upwards of 22,540 HIV-infected children.) The task of the HIV-infected survivor is to learn to live physiologically with the virus that causes acquired immune deficiency syndrome (AIDS) just as he has learned to live with the other seventy or so viruses commonly taking up residence within most human bodies.

Cancer That Comes from Herpes Viruses

Medical science suggests that approximately 30 percent of all cancers are related to viruses. It's also known that about 20 percent of all cancers come from oncogenes, the fifty types of newly discovered special cellular genes found in cancer patients. These gene pieces are part of most individuals' own chromosomes and promote the cancer process. Certain "activating factors" such as, radiation, carcinogenic chemicals, and viruses (e.g. the herpes family of viruses: Epstein-Barr, retrovirus, cytomegalovirus, genital herpes, shingles, HHV-6, and HHV-7) cause oncogenes to become active and to initiate the manufacture of particular proteins, which cause normal cells to turn cancerous.

Just as it's appropriate to avoid exposure to radiation and carcinogens in food, it's best to keep viruses out of one's body or to kill them quickly if they invade. A major means of preventing cancer as well as the symptoms of a viral infection is to take preventive measures against the invasion of viruses. For cancer, the reason is clear: Oncogenes are pieces of viral genes which begin the alteration of human cells and cause them to go into extreme mitotic division. When such excessive mitosis takes place, that's cancer!

There are sixty-three different herpes viruses that cause diseases of various kinds, existing in fish, snakes, oysters, frogs, fungi, birds, rodents, monkeys, household pets, and humans. Seven or more of them are common to people and furnish the potential environment for turning infected cells into mitotic growth factories—malignant tumors.

The Seven Known Herpes Viruses

Since the Roman Emperor Tiberius tried to stop an epidemic 2,000 years ago by outlawing kissing in public places, the herpes virus has been known to have plagued the human race. The name *herpes* comes from the Greek verb *herpein,* which means "to creep."

Herpes simplex virus (HSV) is recognized as having two types, herpes simplex virus type I (HSV-1), associated with diseases of the lips or eyes, and herpes simplex virus type II (HSV-2), genital herpes. Both are transmitted by direct physical contact with a sore on the infected person.

Cytomegalovirus (CMV) is a herpes infection without terribly severe symptoms. CMV, along with the Epstein-Barr virus, is often the source of chronic fatigue syndrome. CMV is spread through the virus's presence in fluid excretions—semen, urine, saliva, breast milk, cervical liquids, and feces—of infected persons.[5]

Epstein-Barr Virus (EBV), once thought to be infectious mononucleosis, is characterized by slow-developing headache, chronic fatigue, chills, sore throat, swollen lymph glands, high fever (up to 105°F), and muscle ache. EBV has been called "the kissing disease" because of its frequent transmission this way; therefore it might be considered as a STD.

Varicella-Zoster Virus (VZ), also known as *herpes zoster,* causes the disease commonly referred to as "shingles." As stated before, chicken pox, derived from this viral infection, lingers as a latent infection and may become active in adult years in the form of shingles sores or blisters and localized pain along the course of sensory nerves. The shingles lesions often are preceded by three days of fever and burning or irritation of the skin. Herpes zoster symptoms are more likely to occur in people who are immunosuppressed.

Human Herpesvirus type VI (HHV-6), discovered relatively recently by Robert Gallo, M.D., of the National Institutes of Health (NIH), was first identified as the African Swine Fever Virus (ASFV). It's divided into two strains, A and B, and HHV-6A is a complicating factor in AIDS (see Chapter 8).[6]

A majority of all the populations living in Western industrialized nations possesses antibodies to HHV-6, meaning that most people in these countries have sustained infections from it.[7] Since the organism can be isolated from saliva, this virus probably is transmitted (like EBV) by coughing, kissing, and other forms of contact with upper respiratory tract secretions.[8] Up to 92 percent of all healthy adults shed the virus in their saliva, so that when somebody sneezes on you, it's more than likely that HHV-6 has been transferred to your respiratory system.

Human Herpesvirus type VII (HHV-7) has joined the other herpes viruses. Isolated as a follow-up to the discovery of human herpesvirus type VI, HHV-7 is little studied and little understood. Like the other herpesviruses, HHV-7 is spread by person-to-person contact; indeed, almost everyone is infected with this virus.

The human herpesviruses (including the neurotropic herpesvirus HSV-1, HSV-2, and varicella-zoster virus, plus the abovementioned group of lymphotropic herpesviruses (EBV, CMV, HHV-6, and HHV-7) have developed a complex set of interactions with their host human beings.[9] They have found a way to infect and remain with us for a lifetime, evading our immune defenses and evolving complex mechanisms for reactivation when our immune defenses become suppressed.

To illustrate how the herpesviruses lie dormant until our immune abilities alter, look at a study conducted by researchers within the Department of Pediatrics at Osaka University Medical School in Osaka, Japan. Human herpesvirus VII was isolated from blood cells of two infants who had typical lesions of roseola (exanthem subitum). The babies had become infected from their mothers *in utero* (through transfer of nourishment during placental feeding). One patient underwent two independent episodes of roseola over the short period of just two months, and both HHV-6 and HHV-7 were then isolated from the child and viewed under the microscope.

The same Osaka investigators tested fifteen additional babies for antibodies to HHV-6 and HHV-7 by the immunofluorescence antibody test. Five of these little patients showed conversion in their blood sera to HHV-7, indicating that this organism is a co-causative agent of roseola. Thus, the mothers were probable sources of their children's infections from some immunodepression they had encountered during the course of their pregnancies.[10]

Calcium Elenolate Kills the Herpes Virus

In 1969, Harold E. Renis, Ph.D., a virologist with The Upjohn Company of Kalamazoo, Michigan, proved that calcium elenolate, an acid-hydrolyzed aqueous extract of elenolic acid, a compound of oleuropein in the olive leaf, is virucidal for all viruses against which it was tested. In particular, Dr. Renis showed that calcium elenolate kills the herpes Virus, including each one known at the time to produce symptoms of a herpes infection: HSV-1, HSV-2, CMV, EBV, and VZ. HHV-6 and HHV-7 had not yet been discovered; HHV-6 was first reported as a disease entity twenty-three years ago and HHV-7 was discovered just three years ago.

Dr. Renis wrote: "We have found calcium elenolate to be virucidal for a broad spectrum of viruses *in vitro* . . . all of the viruses against which calcium elenolate was tested were highly susceptible to inactivation. . . . the virucidal activity of calcium elenolate is mediated through an interaction with the protein coat of the viral particle rather than its nucleic acid."[11]

More than two decades later, the findings of Harold Renis were upheld by three biological scientists working at the Laboratoire de Pharmacognosie, Faculte de Pharmacie, in Rennes, France. They found in 1992 that all of the herpesviruses were inhibited or killed outright by the active antimicrobial ingredients in the plant. As backup to their findings, the three researchers cited in their report twenty-eight references to the virucidal quality of *Olea europeae* L.[12]

CHAPTER 7

ୟ∕୭

How to Eliminate Any Viral Source of Chronic Fatigue Syndrome

Conducting her naturopathic practice in Apex, a suburb of Raleigh, North Carolina, Millie Hinkle, N.D., is truly impressed with the application of olive leaf extract as a germ-inhibiting agent. Dr. Hinkle, who for the past six years has been medical director of the Natural Health Resource Clinic, depends on this antimicrobial herbal agent for patients who are victims of chronic fatigue and immune dysfunction syndrome (CFIDS). Commonly, CFIDS is referred to as "chronic fatigue syndrome" (CFS) by people who have it. Dr. Hinkle administers olive leaf extract for the elimination of yeast infections, protozoa infestations, and in particular, any viral source of chronic fatigue syndrome.

"Two of my patients, each diagnosed with infections of the Epstein-Barr Virus, had been manifesting classical symptoms of chronic fatigue syndrome. They feel wonderfully well when they maintain themselves with olive leaf extract, one capsule three times daily at mealtime. But these CFS suffers don't feel so great if they go off the capsules for any length of time. It's possible that my patients will need to continue to supplement with this product for an indefinite period," Dr. Hinkle says. "Also, literature I've read about the olive leaf extract indicates that a 'die-off' is likely to occur, but my patients have not experienced any. They started in feeling marvelous with elimination of their chronic fatigue syndrome discomforts right from the get-go. That's a good thing.

"In this clinic, my associates and I are putting our patients on olive leaf extract for all kinds of health problems; for infections, of course, but also we're using it to lower blood cholesterol, conquer heart problems, reduce high blood pressure, and treat other troubles. To this point, we have enjoyed its treatment responses for four months. I'm hearing great things about the product from colleagues too— nothing negative whatsoever. I heartily recommend olive leaf extract to others, and absolutely confirm that we in this clinic will continue to use it for our patients," assures Dr. Millie Hinkle.

The Infecting Microbes of Chronic Fatigue Syndrome

Almost invariably, someone suffering from chronic fatigue and immune dysfunction syndrome will be infected with a variety of opportunistic microbes. The invading organisms may include herpesviruses and retroviruses, a certain yeast, and particular parasites, all attracted to the human host by his or her lack of defenses due to a suppressed immune system.

Usually a victim of chronic fatigue syndrome will be affected by an overgrowth of the *Candida albicans* yeast organism. The infesting parasites often consist of protozoa but occasionally helminth worms (usually flukes) are present as well. Most energy-draining and devastating to the psyche, however, are the viral infections connected to CFIDS. Invasion by one or more of the family of viruses—frequently from the herpes group—has been confirmed by numerous health professionals who actively employ olive leaf extract as a therapeutic modality for the chronic fatigue and immune dysfunction condition and its concomitant difficulty, fibromyalgia. Both fibromyalgia (connective tissue pain) and chronic fatigue syndrome respond well to therapy with capsules, tablets, or powdered bulk olive leaf extract.

Elimination of Chronic Fatigue with a Resurgence of Energy

From Scottsdale, Arizona, biochemist Arnold Takemoto, B.S., who designs patient nutritional programs for physicians throughout Arizona, has found olive leaf extract to be an effective addition to his arsenal of natural healing remedies. He has been developing protocols employing methods of complementary medicine for the last sixteen years.

"Olive leaf extract certainly has power, particularly against undesirable microorganisms that are more tenacious. It fills a hole by offering a new and effective tool," says Mr. Takemoto. "I work with a rheumatologist, Lisa Weinrib, M.D., who treats fibromyalgia and chronic fatigue syndrome. Dr. Weinrib has noticed that patients with these problems exhibit much improvement from use of the extract. It's the missing link that functions as an antiviral and antiretroviral agent by slowing down these microorganisms' reproductive cycles. A slowdown of the microbes' spread allows the patient's immune system to go on the attack.

"I have yet to discover another herbal substance that accomplishes antimicrobially what olive leaf extract achieves. During my research for natural remedies, I stumbled on the olive leaf extract and employed it for my daughter. She had just graduated from a school in England and returned home to Phoenix with really severe flu-like symptoms—sore throat, cough, fever, muscular pains, and weakness. She felt awful, came down with chronic fatigue syndrome, and in no way acted like her usual ebullient self," explains Mr. Takemoto. "I put her on the olive leaf extract right away. At first she went through hot and cold sweats, total weariness, debilitation, and other symptoms of a 'die-off' period from the viral, bacterial, fungal, and/or parasitic organisms being killed by the product. But by the end of three days, she suddenly dropped all of her die-off discomforts and gained an immense amount of energy. This injection of energy has lasted continuously for many months, to the present time.

"Next, in addition to taking the large quantity of nutritional supplements that are standard for me, I tried the olive leaf extract on myself. I took it for purposes of acquiring energy. After experiencing one day of die-off, the extract so stimulated my energy level, for days on end it kept me awake working until one o'clock in the morning," Mr. Takemoto says. "My sense is that no single particular intrinsic factor in olive leaf extract gives it efficacy for a variety of uses. In the Bible, the olive tree is named 'the tree of life,' and it furnished a new life of energy for me. Its biological power appears to be in the leaves rather than in the fruit."

EBV as the Main Source of Chronic Fatigue Syndrome

Chronic *Epstein-Barr virus* (EBV) is one of the several viral infections capable of producing the signs and symptoms of chronic fatigue syndrome. Until now, once a person came down with this mononucleosis-like syndrome, there had seldom been any permanent cure. EBV lingers and lies dormant in the body until the individual's immune system again becomes so suppressed that the virus can manifest itself with symptoms, a circumstance described in the prior chapter. The underlying cause of EBV infection has been identified. The synthetically produced environment in which we live in modern society is the reason for such immune suppression.[1]

You already know that Epstein-Barr virus is a member

of the herpes group of viruses. You also know that a common quality of this group of microorganisms is their ability to establish a lifelong latent infection in the human host after the initial infection. For EBV, the latent infection is established owing to lifelong, persistent invasion by the virus of a person's B-lymphocytes (the B-cells) and salivary glands. This latent infection is usually kept in check by the body's highly sophisticated immune surveillance mechanisms. When the human host's immune system is compromised in any way, the latent infection can become active as viral replication and then viral spread are increased. This situation is commonly observed with almost any herpesvirus infection in acquired immune deficiency syndrome (AIDS), cancer, and in drug-induced immunocompromised patients.[2]

Infection with EBV is inevitable among humans. Virtually all persons in the third world, all who are economically disadvantaged, and those living within the confines of ghettos and other crowded parts of the inner city are infected in early adolescence. In middle and upper socioeconomic groups, only about 55 percent of these people have detectable EBV antibodies during adolescence and at the time of entry into college. By the end of early adulthood, however, almost all individuals demonstrate detectable EBV antibodies.[3]

When the primary infection occurs in childhood, it's asymptomatic, but when it occurs in adolescence or early adulthood, the clinical manifestations of infectious mononucleosis (IM) develop in approximately half of the infected people. Transmission or shedding of the virus occurs mainly through saliva during close contact (kissing) and the exchange of other body fluids (sexual intercourse). Expectorating on the street or in buildings leaves droplets of saliva floating in the air which act as sources of airborne infection for people living in close proximity to each other. (Laws against spitting in public places should be enforced vigorously with severe penalties imposed for it.)

Virus shedding in the saliva can continue for two to six months after the initial symptoms of the acute disease have subsided in up to 90 percent of infected persons. In addition, about 20 percent of asymptomatic seropositive (EBV in their blood) adults are shedding virus at any one time and are considered the reservoir for infection among the populace. The rate of EBV shedding is 30 percent higher in the immunosuppressed.[4]

The prolonged carrier state following clinical infectious mononucleosis coupled with the high rate of virus shedding in multimillions of asymptomatic and immunocompromised adults are the major reasons why EBV is so ubiquitous and why CFIDS is exceedingly prevalent.[5]

Diseases Associated with Chronic EBV Syndrome

It has been only within the last decade that sufficient evidence accumulated to implicate Epstein-Barr virus in the broad clinical spectrum of chronic fatigue and associated symptoms of immune dysfunction. Several studies have demonstrated persistently elevated levels of serum antibodies against the early antigen (EA) and viral capsid antigen (VCA) of EBV in a number of patients presenting themselves to doctors with varying combinations of symptoms consistent with this syndrome.

Diseases associated with EBV are shadows of cellular and molecular events that begin with the infection of certain types of epithelial cells, such as those that make up the skin and its related tissues, particularly in the mouth, the pharynx, and the parotid duct. Epithelial cells are the seat of acute infection, and they are shed by the replicating virus, causing inflammation of the throat during infectious mononucleosis and depositing virus in the saliva. EBV reproduces itself within a woman's cervical epithelium as well. In the immune system's B-cells, EBV produces latent infection and proliferation rather than shedding. Thus, different diseases can arise from derangements of either epithelial or lymphoid cells anywhere in the body.[6]

In the thirty years since the discovery of the EBV infection in a Ugandan child with Burkitt's lymphoma (a cancer of the lymphatic system), the virus has been associated with an array of disorders, both benign and malignant. Cellular or molecular "snapshots" allow medical scientists to see that diseases such as hairy leukoplakia, mononucleosis, nasopharyngeal carcinoma, Hodgkin's disease, T-cell lymphoma, parotid carcinoma, all of the different herpes infections, and post-transplantation lymphoma have much in common. Chronic fatigue is their overriding symptom complex.

EBV has adapted to the human species in a variety of ways, usually remaining latent but sometimes destroying cells, occasionally stimulating cells, and eventually evoking immunopathologic reactions in places around the body that are surprising to behold. The panoply of diseases is as varied as the cellular and molecular pathobiology of EBV infection.[7]

Retrovirus as a Cause of CFIDS

There is a recently discovered category of viruses variously designated by virologists as "submicroscopic hijackers," "pirates of the cell," or "pieces of bad news wrapped up in protein." These organisms belong to the viral family known as the *retroviridae* or *retroviruses*. They exhibit persistent pathologies manifesting as debilitating fatigue and flu-like afflictions, and the retroviruses are suspected as being partially responsible for CFIDS.

TABLE 5

Clinical Findings in the Disease Complex of Chronic Fatigue Syndrome or Chronic Fatigue and Immune Dysfunction Syndrome or Chronic Epstein-Barr Virus Syndrome or Chronic Mononucleosis-like Syndrome

(all identifying labels are for the same set of signs and symptoms)

A. FATIGUE
  1. The chief complaint is disabling fatigue which at its worst causes the patient to become totally bedridden.
    a. When bedridden: the patient can do virtually nothing, not even go to the bathroom.
    b. As a shut-in: the patient cannot perform any light housework or its equivalent.
    c. Outside the home: the patient can do all the things usually necessary for home and work, but is more easily fatigued; no energy left for anything else.
  2. Frequency of fatigue:
    a. Consistent and unchanging.
    b. Always some fatigue that may become better but never goes away completely.
    c. The fatigue alternates with feeling normal.
B. PHARYNGITIS (sore throat)—recurrent.
C. MUSCLE ACHES (Myalgia)—recurrent.
  1. The patient needs to stop all normal activities and rest.
  2. The patient can continue normal activities but muscle aches make it difficult.
  3. The patient is not aware of muscle aches during normal activities, only at rest.
D. HEADACHES—recurrent.
  1. The patient needs to stop all normal activities and rest.
  2. The patient can continue normal activities but headaches make it difficult.
  3. The patient is not aware of headaches during normal activities, only at rest.
E. DEPRESSION or unusual mood changes.

F. INSOMNIA
G. LACK OF CONCENTRATION
H. ANXIETY
I. NAUSEA
J. SWOLLEN LYMPH GLANDS (lymphadenopathy)
K. STOMACH ACHE (gastrointestinal discomfort)
L. DIARRHEA
M. COUGH
N. RASH
O. ODD SKIN SENSATIONS
P. LOSS OF APPETITE
Q. JOINT PAINS (arthralgia)
R. VOMITING
S. RECURRENT FEVERS AT HOME (above 37.5°C)
T. INTERMITTENT SWELLING OF FINGERS
U. WEIGHT LOSS
V. WEIGHT GAIN
W. STRESS AT HOME OR WORK
X. HAVE SEEN PHYSICIANS FOR THESE PROBLEMS
Y. THOUGHT SYMPTOMS WERE "JUST ALL IN MY HEAD."
Z. PAST HISTORY
  1. Mononucleosis
  2. Oral herpes
  3. Genital herpes
  4. Herpes zoster (shingles)
  5. Allergies (to food or drugs or hay fever)

Source: P. I. Yutsis, and M. Walker. *The Downhill Syndrome: Doctor, Why Am I So Tired and Suffer with So Many Symptoms?* (Garden City Park, NY: Avery Publishing Group, Inc., 1997).

The search for retroviruses heated up in the fall of 1990, as a result of discoveries made by Elaine DeFreitas, Ph.D., a virologist working at the Wistar Institute in Philadelphia. Dr. DeFreitas had linked chronic fatigue and immune depression syndrome to free-floating pieces of ribonucleic acid (RNA) that translate themselves into deoxyribonucleic acid (DNA). Using their own special enzymes, the reverse transcriptases, these retroviruses are able to splice themselves permanently into the chromosomes of human host cells and turn back upon the cells (that's what makes them "retro" or "reversing" or "turning backward"). Toxins that they create disrupt the infected cells and promote disease symptoms.[8]

The Reversal Mechanism of Retroviruses

NIH virologist Robert Gallo, M.D., states: "All retroviruses are very similar in their size, morphology, content, much of their genome [gene strand], and replication cycle. But virologists have been able to subclassify them, based on their observations that, despite common characteristics, the biological effects of retroviruses are diverse."[9]

Researchers have long been intrigued, and a bit unnerved, by the retroviral subfamily of microbes known as spuma or "foamy" viruses. Spuma viruses are described as foamy because they induce extensive fluid-filled spaces (vacuolization) within the host cells that they infect.

W. John Martin, M.D., Ph.D., chief of molecular immunopathology at the University of Southern California Medical Center, Los Angeles, has linked the mysterious foamy retrovirus to the enigmatic symptoms of chronic fatigue syndrome. Dr. Martin found foamy retroviruses in almost all patients with this disease. They exhibited typically persistent, debilitating, flulike symptoms, exactly as experienced by those people complaining of CFIDS.

Many people afflicted with chronic fatigue syndrome suffer unexplained neurological problems. Until Martin's research, the spumaviruses hadn't been linked to human disease.[10]

Four separate research teams have confirmed Dr. Martin's findings by uncovering the foamy viral infection among patients with CFIDS. Now both Dr. Martin and Dr. DeFreitas, in separate investigations, have succeeded in extracting whole human foamy viruses from patients showing symptoms of chronic fatigue syndrome.

Dr. Martin found evidence of the virus in 160 out of 300

patients diagnosed with chronic fatigue syndrome—some of whose symptoms were not so serious. He has been studying CFIDS since 1988 when local specialists started sending him patients with strange brain conditions.[11]

Since late fall 1990, Dr. Martin and Dr. DeFreitas, in their separate laboratories, have both succeeded at extracting a whole virus—not just a genetic marker—from patients suffering with chronic fatigue syndrome. Dr. Martin cites three reasons for attributing symptoms of brain dysfunction to the foamy virus.

First, he says, it looks like a foamy virus; viewed through an electron microscope, the virus has a spherical outer coat and resides mainly in vacuoles, or pockets, in the cytoplasm of cells.

Second, it acts like a foamy virus, making cultured cells swell and stick together in large foamy masses.

Third, it reacts to probes made from the simian (monkey) foamy virus, a relative of human foamy virus (HFV).

Is Another Retrovirus Possibly Causing CFIDS?

Once called chronic Epstein-Barr virus syndrome, much finger-pointing at other viral organisms either joining with or substituting for EBV has forced a name change. Dr. Elaine DeFreitas is investigating HTLV-2, Dr. John Martin is focused on the spumavirus, Peter Behan, M.D., of the University of Glasgow in Scotland, is studying enteroviruses that include the polio virus, and Dr. Anthony L. Komaroff at Boston's Women's and Brigham Hospital has been investigating the cytomegalovirus and the human herpesvirus type VI.

These kinds of infectious viruses already reside in most people but are held at bay by their immune systems. But Jay A. Levy, Ph.D., a biomedical researcher working at the University of California in San Francisco, and the principal investigator for a research study published in the British medical journal *Lancet,* has shown that victims of chronic fatigue syndrome possess abnormal immune systems that fail to clear the body of invading viruses or to prevent reactivation of latent ones. Together with Nancy Klimas, Ph.D., another immunologist at the University of Miami School of Medicine, Dr. Levy has raised the question of whether chronic fatigue syndrome patients with failing immune systems are showing the cause or effect of their affliction. Until the remedy of olive leaf extract was uncovered (or rediscovered), there has been only inexact treatment for the viral sources of chronic fatigue syndrome.

Eliminate Any Viral Source of Chronic Fatigue Syndrome

There may be other viral sources of chronic fatigue syndrome besides Epstein-Barr virus and retrovirus. They could include *cytomegalovirus, human herpes virus-VI,* and more. But elimination of the microbe is most important, and each of these organisms responds well to the oral ingestion of olive leaf extract. Sufficient quantities of this olive leaf–derived food supplement, swallowed daily in repeated doses, gets rid of the disease symptoms of chronic fatigue syndrome. Eradication of microbial causes of CFIDS happens, quite simply, from the nontoxic hydrolyzed components, elenolic acid with its calcium elenolate salt, bound by nature into the leaf structure.

The virucidal effect of calcium elenolate has an affinity for thirteen or more specific viruses or virus families (i.e. the seven herpes viruses) which are listed in Table 6. Inasmuch as retroviruses were not discovered until the current decade, they are not included in the table created from research done in 1969 and 1970, by the Department of Virology Research of The Upjohn Company.

The virucidal activity *in vitro* and *in vivo* of this olive leaf compound was shown to be greatest under alkaline

TABLE 6

Spectrum of Virucidal Activity of Calcium Elenolate

(Calcium elenolate 1 mg/ml was incubated with an equal volume of virus suspension at 37°C for 30 minutes to discover the virucidal effect)

The Incubated Viruses Killed by Calcium Elenolate

- Herpesviruses (all species)
- Vaccinia
- Pseudorabies
- Newcastle Disease
- Parainfluenza Virus 3
- Coxsackie Virus A21
- Encephalomyocarditis
- Polio Virus 1
- Polio Virus 2
- Polio Virus 3
- Vesicular Stomatitis
- Sinbis Virus
- Reovirus 3

Source: H. E. Renis, "In vitro antiviral activity of calcium elenolate." *Antimicrobial Agents and Chemotherapy* 167–172, 1970.

conditions at a pH of 7.5. The quantity of virus inactivated by The Upjohn Company was dependent on the calcium elenolate concentration and the time of incubation. When the incubation of calcium elenolate was carried out with amino acids prior to incubation with any of the viruses, losses in virucidal activity were detected with the amino acids glycine, lysine, cysteine, and histidine, and to a lesser extent with phenylalanine, tryptophan, serine, and threonine.

The company scientists stated: "We have found calcium elenolate to be virucidal for a broad spectrum of viruses in vitrol, to reduce virus yields from hamsters infected with parainfluenza 3 virus, and to have a low order of toxicity after intranasal instillation."[12]

❧

CHAPTER 8

Changing HIV Positive (+) Blood to HIV Negative (-)

Though poorly understood, there probably already exist adequate immune mechanisms within the human body to control, possibly even eliminate, the virus thought to cause a complex of diseases known as *acquired immunodeficiency syndrome,* or *AIDS.*[1] Described in this chapter are recipes for a self-formulated drink, tea, and herbal, to reverse pathological blood factors, possibly changing them from HIV positive (+) to HIV negative (-). My information is taken from interviews, published reports, anecdotes, trials, and testings undertaken by members of the AIDS-support organization Keep Hope Alive of West Allis, Wisconsin, under the executive directorship of Mark Konlee.

From 1981, when the first individuals who exhibited extreme immune system suppression were discovered in Los Angeles, followed by isolation of the human immunodeficiency virus (HIV) by French scientists in 1983, acquired immunodeficiency syndrome has been a puzzling and death-dealing disease. AIDS and HIV are no less controversial today than they were two-and-a-half decades ago. HIV, the virus cited by a majority of scientists to be the source of AIDS (a conclusion disputed by some of the militant groups representing *p*eople *w*ith AIDS [PWAs]), continues to yield conflicting and unpredictable data. Medical researchers and clinicians are trying unsuccessfully to cope with this virus and its associated disease, but their efforts are generating more questions than answers.

Most often organizations speaking on behalf of PWAs are at odds with the treatment approaches advocated by the allopathic medical community. Most PWA political groups accuse mainstream AIDS researchers and the pharmaceutical companies who sponsor them of using people with AIDS as so many human "guinea pigs." Growing out of these long-standing differences, natural substances and drugs are distributed through underground pharmacies or "buyers' clubs," which acquire remedies from places like South America, Europe, Asia, and Israel.[2]

Buyers' clubs catering to people with AIDS operate in a twilight zone, somewhere between a licensed drugstore and a pharmaceutical Casbah. (See the Appendix for the names and addresses of sources of information or products.) Almost all buyers' clubs also sell vitamins, minerals, and other over-the-counter health care products at bargain prices. But their principal business is dispensing remedies that are otherwise unavailable in the allopathic drug marketplace. They *do* earn a living from their endeavors, but the proprietors of these buyers' clubs offer their services mostly out of a sense of compassion.[3]

Keep Hope Alive seems not to be a buyers' club, and does not sell products except subscriptions to its newsletter. My interview with Mark Konlee left me with the distinct impression that he cares deeply about AIDS victims and those who are HIV positive.

The Disbelief That HIV Causes AIDS

The current belief among allopathic medical doctors and infectious disease specialists is that HIV destroys a subgroup of lymphocytes in the blood, resulting in suppression of the body's immune response—AIDS. Acute infecton following exposure to the virus results in the production of certain antibodies (by seroconversion). The presence of antibodies indicates that infection has taken place; however, not all those persons who seroconvert progress to chronic infection.

For patients who do enter a chronic stage of infection, there may be illness of varying severity, including persistent generalized involvement of the lymph nodes; what is termed *AIDS-related complex (ARC)* with symptoms of intermittent fever, weight loss, diarrhea, fatigue, and night sweats; and AIDS itself, presented to victims as opportunistic infections, especially pneumonia caused by the protozoan *Pneumocystis carinii* and/or tumors, such as Kaposi's sarcoma.

Although HIV has been isolated from semen, cervical secretions, plasma, cerebrospinal fluid, tears, saliva, urine, and breast milk, the HIV concentration shows wide variations. Mark Konlee, editor/publisher of *Positive Health News,* and his 20,000 subscribers hold with another belief. They say the real culprit causing AIDS is the human herpesvirus type VI, strain A (HHV-6A). And Keep Hope Alive members add, HIV becomes dangerous only in the presence of HHV-6A,[4] and HIV is a fragile virus that does not survive well outside the body. Still, even in the face of such fragility, AIDS is pandemic, and until now, there has been no known cure.

Peter Duesberg, M.D., considered one of the most eminent virologists in the United States—the first scientist to sequence the genetic code of a retrovirus—has repeatedly questioned HIV as the cause of AIDS.[5] Other notable scientists, such as Karry Mullis, M.D., Nobel laureate and inventor of the polymerase chain reaction (PCR), the most sensitive method of detecting and isolating the human immunodeficiency virus, also question HIV as the sole cause of AIDS. In fact, Dr. Mullis and Dr. Duesburg are among the 300+ researchers who belong to Scientists for the Scientific Reappraisal of the HIV/AIDS Hypothesis (SSRHAH). The

SSRHAH position, based on compelling data in biology and epidemiology, showing repeated inconsistencies and contradictions regarding the HIV/AIDS connection, is that HIV could not possibly cause AIDS on its own, and is probably more like a viral hitchhiker along for the ride.[6]

Reported Benefits from Using Olive Leaf Extract for AIDS

Practicing family medicine in Covina, California, James Robert Privitera, Jr., M.D., is credited by Mark Konlee with discovering that a concentrate of olive leaves, containing natural protease inhibitors, used in combination with the immune modulator Naltrexone, both dissolved in a whole lemon/olive oil drink, has reduced the human immunodeficiency virus (HIV) viral load from a high count of 58,000 to nondetectable blood levels in two weeks. With results for HIV patients who use olive leaf extract confirmed by their undergoing the ELISA/Western Blot blood tests, the patients' HIV antibody status changes from positive to negative.

The discovery of lessened HIV antibodies resulting from an HIV patient taking olive leaf extract occurred in August 1995. At the same time, the laboratory examining the patient's blood reported that it observed his blood cell counts increasing in immunoability with greater numbers of CD^4 and CD^8 lymphocytes.

Have you wondered about what the "CD" references mean as they relate to one's immune status? Here is the definition of CD: A uniform system of nomenclature has been adopted by scientists who have as their medical specialty immunology and/or hematology. For these specialists, all cell surface molecules on the outer surfaces of lymphocytes (the T-cells and B-cells) act as markers. Such cell surface markers are assigned the letters "CD," which designates the *cluster determinant*. This

CD is followed by a number indicating the sequence of acceptance of antigens with which antibodies react, added to this as part of the number is the order of discovery of the marker cell. Thus CD^4 or CD^8 indicates the sequence of cell surface proteins on a certain kind of lymphocyte and when the proteins were found. To date, the numbered sequence of proteins on lymphocytes goes up to CD^{78}. However, the *function* of only a few cell surface markers have been adequately determined.[7]

Olive Leaf Extract Contains Protease Inhibitors

In *Positive Health News,* Mark Konlee writes: "Protease inhibitors are rapidly bringing new hope and breathing new life into people with AIDS (PWAs) long exhausted by azidothymidine (AZT) monotherapy."[8] Protease inhibitors are substances that stop the action of enzymes which, responding to toxins from the human immunodeficiency virus, break down tissue protein that makes up the muscles, ligaments, skin, and other components of one's body.

Discovered by the community of PWAs in the spring of 1996 is a natural source of protease inhibitors coming from olive leaf extract that's available over the counter and without prescription. When this olive leaf extract is combined with the immune modulator Naltrexone and a drink made from lemon juice and olive oil, it has produced stunning results for PWAs. Their viral loads tend to drop to nondetectable levels in just two to four weeks.

In the first test case ever recorded of an AIDS patient who used olive leaf extract therapeutically—identified by the initials J. P.—the patient's HIV antibody status changed from positive to negative on both the ELISA and Western Blot standard AIDS tests. The results were confirmed by retesting.

Here's what happened, as reported by Mark Konlee: On

March 3, 1996, J.P. started taking olive leaf extract, one capsule four times a day. For some time before that date, he had been complaining to his friends and doctors of discomfort from swollen lymph nodes, and no drug treatment had been able to shrink them. (*Lymph nodes* are small filters of the lymph fluid that prevent foreign particles from entering the bloodstream. They swell when infection is present.)

From taking the olive leaf extract, the next day, J.P. explained, he felt a significant increase in energy along with a mild headache (probably the die-off reaction). By March seventh, he reported, all his swollen lymph nodes were completely gone. His headache had disappeared as well. By March eighteenth, on his way to a local hospital to have blood drawn for laboratory testing, J.P. stated he had never felt so good nor had so much energy. He said, "I feel twenty years younger."

The laboratory test results were astounding. J.P.'s CD^4 count of 30 (on January 21) had risen to 40. A CD^8 count of 1380 elevated to 1920. He tested negative to the P24 Antigen test. His Western Blot test came out negative. Furthermore, the patient's PCR test by the Roche Amplicor method became undetectable.

(The *PCR* or *polymerase chain reaction* is a technique used in molecular genetics. The DNA of a single cell, treated with polymerase enzymes, replicates many times. This supplies DNA in quantities sufficient to analyze for the identification of viruses and other purposes.)

By April tenth, J.P.'s test results showed that his HIV count remained nondetectable; Beta-2 microglobulin levels stayed at zero; P24 Antigen was at zero; ELISA and Western Blot HIV Antibody tests both showed negative; HHV-6 in the blood was nondetectable; and his CD^4 count rose to 114.

His physician, highly experienced in treating AIDS patients, told J.P. that never before in her career had she seen a set of lab results like this from an AIDS patient. From the laboratory readings, J.P. might be considered to no longer have AIDS.

A Second HIV Test Case Benefits from the Olive Leaf

A second HIV test case reported by Mark Konlee in *Positive Health News* was that of C.D. C.D. used the combination of Naltrexone, the whole lemon/olive oil drink and olive leaf extract, which reduced his viral load from an exceedingly elevated 160,000 organisms per milliliter of blood down to 30,000 in two weeks, and then dropped it to 692 in eleven weeks. A fall in viral load this dramatic has never been achieved from the use of AZT.

Additionally, after finishing a second bottle of olive leaf extract (120 capsules in all), two of the three lesions from Kaposi's sarcoma showing on his chest had disappeared. (*Kaposi's sarcoma* [*KS*] is a slowly evolving malignant tumor arising from blood vessels in the skin and appearing as purple to dark brown plaques or nodules which may be one of the complications of AIDS.)

Four more PWAs responded to the olive leaf drink combination, too. Their experiences took place throughout the summer and into the fall of 1996. The positive experiences for PWAs have continued, and statistical information is now being gathered by Keep Hope Alive for a presentation to the AIDS community nationwide.

Olive Leaf Extract Used Alone as AIDS Treatment

Using four capsules per day of olive leaf extract over a period of approximately fifteen weeks, case number seven had a somewhat lessened reaction to the herbal remedy. The HIV + patient's viral load dropped from 37,000 to 19,500 in those three-and-a-half months, which is equivalent to the response of a person with AIDS taking AZT for the first time, when the most dramatic drop in viral load usually takes place.

But this case showed something more in therapeutic progress that was highly encouraging. He had increases in his CD^4, from 239 to 296; CD^8 elevated from 288 to 365; and his white blood cell count rose from 2100 to 2900—a marked boost of his immune system had occurred.

Another PWA added capsules of olive leaf extract alone to his standard treatment protocol. He takes the capsules as a monotherapy, without drinking the whole lemon/olive oil cocktail, and sees improvement. Still, Mark Konlee strongly recommends that olive leaf extract be taken in conjunction with Naltrexone and the daily use of a whole lemon/olive oil drink. Also, Mark offers a recipe for brewing your own olive leaf extract tea using unadulterated olive leaves. Additional information is given below.

Recipe for the Whole Lemon/Olive Oil Drink

Nearly all of the PWAs cited above who benefited from taking olive leaf extract were simultaneously drinking a mixture of whole lemon and olive oil. What follows is the recipe for blending a whole lemon/olive oil drink to be taken with olive leaf extract and other items.[9]

1. Cut up one medium lemon into quarters. Put the whole fruit, including the rind and seeds, in a blender. (For a less bitter drink, squeeze in the juice of a whole lemon and blend in the rind of one-half lemon.)
2. You may add one-and-a-half cups of orange juice, other fruit juice, or water to make the mixture more palatable.
3. Add one tablespoon of cold pressed extra virgin olive oil.
4. Blend the ingredients together at high speed for two minutes.
5. Filter the mixture through a strainer to separate the juice

from the pulp. Discard the pulp and drink the remaining liquid, either all at once with olive leaf extract capsules, or divide into two or three daily portions.

How to Make Anti-AIDS Olive Leaf Tea

Leaves from the olive tree for brewing into tea may be acquired from one particular source in the United States known to me (see the Appendix). Be aware that these leaves are likely to be imported from countries such as Turkey and Greece, where the leaves may not be handled in the best manner. First, they will be sprayed with copper sulphate, which is not recommended for human consumption because it's toxic. Second, they are whacked off tree branches by pickers using long sticks. Such leaves will probably contain breaks, cuts, and other flaws, which tend to oxidize, especially during the long overseas trip aboard slow transport ships. Consequently, certain batches of leaves will have less elenolic acid, calcium elenolate, and other hydrolysis products, and a subsequent loss of potency. The best possible leaves to purchase would be those growing on manzanillo olive trees in Southern Calfiornia, though most are processed into olive leaf extract.

What follows are the preparations for a recipe from Keep Hope Alive for brewing your own anti-AIDS olive leaf tea to drink three times a day:

Preparations for Brewing Olive Leaf Tea

1. Buy a one-pound bag of whole olive leaves that have been air dried at temperatures not exceeding 150°F. Ask your whole olive leaf supplier to advise you of the drying temperature level for the leaves you are purchasing; drying at higher temperature will destroy much of the leaves' antimicrobial components.
2. Use one-half of the olive leaves (1/2 pound) for brewing. Store the balance of leaves in a plastic bag at

room temperature for brewing into the next batch when you're ready to do so.

3. Have available one gallon of distilled water or spring water.
4. Be prepared with a five- or six-quart crock pot.
5. Have on hand at least two glass bottles of about two-quart capacity, so as to hold three-and-a-half quarts of brewed tea.
6. Have a candy-making thermometer handy.

Recipe for Brewing Olive Leaf Tea

Place one-half pound (eight ounces) of whole olive leaves in a bowl and rinse away impurities by adding enough purified water to cover the leaves. Drain the water. Add the olive leaves to your crock pot and fill it with one gallon of distilled or spring water. Cover the crock pot and set on the stove.

Turn the stove heat to low and let the water simmer. After six hours, check the temperature with a candy thermometer. The ideal temperature range is between 175°F and 185°F. Keep the water heating, checking hourly, until it reaches this range. When you've reached the target temperature, move the pot cover off center by about one-quarter inch, so some heat escapes. Because moisture will also escape, after ten hours, add enough water to bring the liquid up to its original one-gallon level. Replace the cover tightly.

Keep checking the temperature hourly to maintain it at the 175°F–185°F range. After it has simmered for twelve hours, turn off the heat and allow the crock pot to cool to room temperature, for from four to six hours. Then, using a cup, scoop out several four-ounce cups of olive leaf tea and place them in glass bottles for later use. Pour the balance of the liquid through a strainer to remove the leaves. Discard the leaves, since you should not use them again for brewing. Refrigerate the tea in closed glass bottles. The strained tea can be used immediately. The unstrained tea may be stored for up to two weeks for later use. Strain before drinking.

Dosage for Taking Olive Leaf Tea

For adults, drink one-half cup of olive leaf tea three times daily to boost immune system response. Slower changes in laboratory test readings occur when the tea is drunk twice daily. Take the tea once in the morning, at noon, and in the late afternoon, but not later than 7:00 P.M. If you drink the olive leaf tea before bedtime, you'll probably experience insomnia from the energy this drink creates. Just like the olive leaf extract, this tea's components are excellent for overcoming chronic fatigue syndrome, a complication often striking PWAs.

To mask the bitter taste associated with olive leaves, you can add plain water, ginger ale or soda water, but never cola drinks (too much caffeine and sugar). You can make iced tea by adding one-half cup of olive leaf tea to a large glass with ice and a slice of lemon.

Successes Reported by PWAs from Drinking Olive Leaf Tea

Case reports dated November 25, 1996, and published by Keep Hope Alive indicate that drinking olive leaf tea improves laboratory test readings. M. reports that his viral load decreased from the highest level of 380,000 to 129,000 in six-and-a-half weeks. He also showed increases in his CD^3, CD^4, CD^8, platelet, and white blood cell counts.

An HIV positive woman, D., says that her viral load fell from a high of 168,000 to 18,000 in three weeks and three days from drinking three one-half cups of olive leaf tea three times daily. As a result, her body temperature increased from a subnormal of 96.4°F to 98.4°F, and her chronically swollen lymph nodes normalized.

All of the information coming from Keep Hope Alive is available in one self-published text, *How to Reverse Immune Dysfunction,* by Mark Konlee, at PO Box 27041, West Allis, Wisconsin 53227.[10]

CHAPTER 9

✿

A Quick Cure for the Common Cold and Flu

Did you know:

    . . . that the common cold is both the most serious and least serious disease affecting people anywhere on earth?

    . . . that the common cold infects 90 percent of the North American population every year?

    . . . that the common cold produces ten times more illness in children than all other diseases combined?

    . . . that the common cold causes up to 120 million lost schooldays and 100 million lost workdays each year?

    . . . that the common cold is the most persistent enemy of good health for humankind?

    . . . that a single sneeze can project 4,500 droplets of a contagious cold- or flu-inducing virus a distance of twelve feet at over 100 miles per hour?

    . . . that once the flu virus enters a community, it attacks as much as one-third of the general community, and more than half the people living in institutions such as boarding schools and nursing homes?

    . . . that the flu virus can live for hours in dried mucus— on doorknobs, telephones, faucets, or wherever flu-infected people with unwashed hands have passed?

... that there was no known cure for the common cold
and flu until the early 1960s when such a cure was
discovered to be present in olive leaves?

The Common Cold in History and Literature

What the average person currently calls "a cold," and
the medical profession refers to as an "upper respiratory
infection," is an ailment assigned various intriguing names
by people throughout history. The common cold has been
identified as "catarrh," "rheum," "coryza," "the miser-
ies," "the sniffles," and other things. Most of these terms
come from classical roots relating to "running" and "steam-
ing," suggesting some of the symptoms of the condition.

Catarrh, for example, comes from the Greek *katarrho*,
meaning to flow. Coryza, also from the Greek, derives from
koruza, literally meaning "running of the nose." Because
in the past so little was known about the common cold and
its causes, some of this terminology was also applied to
other ailments with similar symptoms.

The first reference to the cold as we know it today,
appearing in the *Oxford English Dictionary*, is dated 1537
in the state papers of King Henry VIII. The monarch complains of the problems that may occur "If I take any cold."

Biblical writings recorded in the *Comprehensive Concor-
dance of the Scriptures* fail to show references to ailments
that would suggest the common cold, although in the *Old
Testament*, II Kings, there is a parable of a boy who complains about his head while working in the fields, is taken
home apparently lifeless, is given warmth, and makes a
miraculous sudden recovery signaled by seven sneezes.

Despite the apparent lack of references in the *Concor-
dance*, it seems highly unlikely that people of Biblical times
were lucky enough to escape the curse of the common cold.

Shakespeare's plays contain numerous references to the
ailment both under the old term "rheum" and the current

"cold." For instance, in *King Henry the Fourth, Part Two,* Bullcalf, an army recruit, when asked what ails him, replies bitterly: ". . . a whoreson cold, sir; a cough, sir, which I caught with ringing in the king's affairs upon his coronation, sir."

Grumio, a servant in *The Taming of the Shrew,* complains that the weather is so bad he fears catching cold, and before the scene ends he announces: "I have caught an extreme cold."

Shakespeare's *The Comedy of Errors* has Drumio cautioning, regarding another character, "Let him walk whence he came lest he catch cold on his feet." And references to colds appear in a dozen or more of the Bard's works.

In old usage, according to the *Oxford English Dictionary,* a cold confined mainly to the nose and pharynx was called a "cold in the head." When accompanied by a discharge from the eyes, the term used was a "crying cold." By any other name, a cold is just as miserable as it has always been—no matter the cause.

The Rhinovirus Plagues Us All

The rhinovirus (RV), possibly the most common cause of the common cold, is responsible for more than 40 percent of all cold symptoms. This virus is so small that it must be magnified 400,000 times to be identified by a virologist (see Illustration 9-1). In truth, the rhinovirus is actually a family of more than 120 cold-inducing viruses and can be blamed for most of the 250 colds an average adult suffers during a lifetime. People all over the world catch from 1 to 6 colds a year on average.

RV is not bothered by extremes of cold or heat, and it scorns antibiotics, which are designed to fight bacteria, not viruses. When physicians prescribe antibiotics for cold sufferers, they are doing a disservice not only to their patients, but to all of humanity, by encouraging mutations of pathogenic bacteria, making them antibiotic-resistant. On the other hand, a physician might prescribe an antibiotic for cold symptoms in order to fend off a secondary bacterial infection that could have developed along with the cold.

Still, the cold virus is very definitely killed by taking capsules of olive leaf extract. It's the calcium elenolate hydrolysis product of the oleuropein in olive leaf extract that does it. Renowned virologist M. G. Soret, Ph.D., from the Department of Virology Research, a division of The Upjohn Company, states: "In the search for antiviral drugs, calcium elenolate was found to have *in vitro* activity against a variety of viruses [at least six of them], including several agents of human 'common colds.' As a potential *in vivo* antiviral drug, calcium elenolate was tested in parainfluenza 3 infection of hamsters. These tests mimic the infection, treatment, and sampling procedures employed in 'common cold' studies in human volunteers.'' Incidentally, the calcium elenolate was administered to the hamsters as nasal washings.[2]

The nasal washings worked well, which leaves me with the distinct impression that olive leaf extract made into nose drops would be effective as another method of delivering this quick cure for the common cold.

And this easy-to-take natural therapy for the common cold, available as an over-the-counter nutritional supplement without prescription, is shown to be unquestionably safe. Its safety and efficacy was proven by professor Shalom Z. Hirschman, M.D., during the years 1970 and 1971, while he worked in the Division of Infectious Diseases of the Department of Medicine at the Mount Sinai School of Medicine, the City University of New York.[3]

Dr. Hirschman thought that the virus-killing product he had tested in olive leaves, crystalline calcium elenolate $[`C^{11}H^{13}O^6)^2Ca]$, was so virucidal and safe for use against DNA and RNA viruses, he advocated its administration for inhibiting murine leukemia viruses, those murine viruses that cause the potentially fatal blood dyscrasia, leukemia.[4]

The Exact Description of a Common Cold

Does anyone not have experience with the illness called "the common cold"? It is an upper respiratory viral infection, usually a mild disease that runs its course in seven to ten days. Characteristic symptoms include nasal congestion and discharge, sore throat, headache, and low-grade fever. In nicotine-addicted persons who smoke cigarettes, says Steven Seidenfeld, M.D., fellow in Infectious Diseases in the Department of Medicine at the University of Texas Health Science Center at Dallas, the illness may be more severe and last up to three weeks.

"Smoking governs the course of a common cold significantly, and smokers with colds tend to have more upper and lower respiratory symptoms, and the symptoms persist longer," says John Mills, M.D., the author of an article about how to prevent the common cold, published in *Modern Medicine*. "Industrial studies show that smokers with upper respiratory disease lose considerably more workdays than nonsmokers."[5] If you're addicted to nicotine and smoking, taking olive leaf extract prophylactically on a daily basis to prevent colds and flu is a wise move.

U.S. Frequency of Locations for the Common Cold

The major virus that causes colds, rhinovirus, has two peak activity periods during the year—one around the time school starts in the United States and the other in mid-winter. Fall is when colds infect about one-third of the population as a whole. Just slightly less than another third get their colds in the winter. Somewhat more than one-fifth of Americans contract cold ailments in the spring, while summer brings relative relief to all but 8 percent of the people.

If you live in the northeastern United States, you have

twice as much chance of catching cold as do Americans residing in the South. And you're eight to nine times more susceptible than residents of the west-central and Pacific areas of the country. The distribution of colds throughout the United States is: the Northeast, 47 percent; the East Central region, 17 percent; the West Central area, 6 percent; the South, 25 percent; and the Pacific region, 5 percent.

The rhinovirus gets its name from its favorite port of entry into our bodies. *Rhino* is a Greek prefix referring to the nasal passages. The nose and eyes are RV's main invasion routes into the human physiological system.

How does the rhinovirus get transmitted? The germs causing colds do not get spread around by exposure to low outside temperatures. That's fiction. Actually, many people living in polar-bear climates never experience colds until exposed to infected visitors from other areas, either local or from a distance. Also, the RV isn't necessarily spread around by kissing, for it's seldom found anywhere outside of the nasal fluid. (The eyes are a source of infection since the tear ducts drain into the nose.)

Rather, the true cause for cold virus transmission is direct contact—when a person touches the hands of a cold sufferer, or a contaminated surface, such as a desktop, table, telephone, or doorknob, and then conveys the virus to his eyes or nose. Most of all, colds spread hand to hand (by shaking hands) followed by rubbing one's own eyes or nose.

The cold virus can survive and remain active for up to three days on environmental surfaces. And when RV enters one of your cells, it commands that cell to reproduce more microorganisms just like it, to go about the dirty work of making you miserable.

RV can survive in temperatures as low as minus 200°F. It's killed in human tissues only by something virucidal, like olive leaf extract. Nothing else touches the cold virus. Many physicians practicing wholistic medicine, who are aware of the monoterpene hydrolysis products derived from oleuropein, elenolic acid, and/or calcium elenolate, are now recommending three steps to control the spread of colds by contact: (1) frequent hand washing after direct contact with people who have colds, (2) keeping your own hands from touching the eyes and nose, and (3) daily consumption of a capsule or two or more of olive leaf extract.

Olive Leaf Extract Prevents or Cures "the Flu"

As reported to the American Society for Microbiology in August 1975, "Calcium elenolate inactivates all myxoviruses."[6] Myxoviruses are the germs that cause a lower respiratory tract infection known as "the flu" which may arise from any one of the three different kinds of influenza viruses: types A, B, and C. Type A is the worst, the cause of the pandemic Spanish flu of 1918 (killing 20 million people), the Asian flu of 1957, the Hong Kong flu of 1968, and other epidemics occurring in England (1972), Texas (1977), Bangkok (1979), the Philippines (1982), Mississippi (1985), and Leningrad (1986). There are three different strains, or subtypes, of influenza type A.

Influenza type B causes serious illness, but is not so widespread and has no subtypes. Influenza type C causes only mild illness. Types A and B mutate slightly each year so that different variations do emerge.[7]

Olive leaf extract is effective against all types and strains of "the flu" and all other viruses causing lower respiratory tract infections. If you take prophylactic doses of this food supplement, you probably won't be a candidate for infection by the influenza types A, B, or C, if your immune system is working decently. Yet, bacterial pneumonia may occur from any trace of an influenza viral invasion; therefore, I am in no way suggesting avoidance of a yearly vaccination with the currently prevalent strain of influenza virus. Such a vaccination is especially necessary for the high-risk population, such as the fragile elderly, the very young, those with chronic diseases of the lungs, and other debilitated persons affected by cancer, heart ailments, or other degenerative diseases.

If you're otherwise in good health, and take olive leaf extract daily, you aren't likely to experience the onset of symptoms of "the flu" which consist of sore throat, cough, fever, muscular pains, chills, general discomfort, and weakness. The incubation period lasts from one to three days, and the symptoms usually strike suddenly. Only the fever and nonlocal symptoms distinguish this lower respiratory tract infection we call "the flu" from the common cold, which is strictly an upper respiratory tract infection.

That the calcium elenolate present in olive leaf extract is a quick cure for "the flu" was proven by a 1977 report published in the *Archives of Virology*. This natural food supplement, investigated as a drug, was then administered by the biologist researcher as nose drops to hamsters he had inoculated with the influenza virus, strain A (the most dangerous type). The animals were cured quickly. The biologist summarized his research when he wrote: "Calcium elenolate, a virucidal agent, reduced the virus titers of nasal washes when the drug was given as nose drops near the time of virus inoculation so as to affect high drug concentrations in the nasal passages."[8]

Correction for the Other Lower Respiratory Tract Infections

Ben Z. Katz, M.D., Associate Professor of Pediatrics, Northwestern University Medical School, and Richard B. Thomson, Jr., Ph.D., Director of Microbiology and Virology in the Department of Pathology and Laboratory Medicine of Evanston Hospital in Evanston, Illinois, point out that "the flu" comes from the influenza virus and is one of the group of lower respiratory tract infections represented as well by croup (acute laryngotracheaobronchitis) from infection with the parainfluenza virus infection, bronchiolitis, and pneumonia of viral origin.[9]

Influenza organisms are the only members of the Orthomyxoviridae family, against which calcium elenolate in olive leaf extract has proven efficacious as a virucidal. It's also used effectively to prevent or kill off an existing infection with the parainfluenza viruses that cause croup, bronchiol disease, and viral pneumonia.

Viral pneumonia can complicate an infection caused by the type A influenza virus, but olive leaf extract is useful as treatment for both conditions. At any pH, its calcium elenolate inactivates the infectivity of the myxoviruses, including influenza virus type A, the Newcastle disease virus (NDV), and the parainfluenza type 3 in an administered strength of 0.25 mg per ml.[10]

Calcium elenolate also works well against coxsackievirus, the cause of hand-foot-mouth syndrome, a mild illness affecting young children, manifested by mouth ulcers and painful blisters on the hands and feet.[11] It works great to bring about a cure for an adult who has the mumps, too.

The Chiropractor Who Cured Her Mumps with Calcium Elenolate

Penelope Roberts, D.C., age forty-nine, a practicing chiropractor in Carbondale, Colorado, took olive leaf extract to quickly cure her adult-onset mumps after all other natural therapies had failed. Being an enthusiastic chiropractor, Dr. Roberts would never dream of using drugs or other types of allopathic treatment. She had gone through a severe bout of facial infection, which she at first believed came from dental work, but it hadn't. Her symptoms started on November 28, 1996, three days after her visit to the dentist. All signs and symptoms of her mumps were gone by December seventh.

The mumps, a childhood disease that's dangerous when

it strikes adults, is caused by a member of the family of viruses known as *paramyxoviridae*. It invades and multiplies in the parotid gland but is attracted to all glands and nerves in the body. The mumps is being described, as a conclusion to this chapter about the "common cold" and "the flu," because it's a respiratory virus, like those other two diseases transferred by direct contact. The virus can travel a few feet suspended in air droplets from a mumps victim's cough or sneeze. It is the second most common cause of viral meningitis.[12]

Dr. Penelope Roberts, of course, comes in direct contact with patients when she lays hands on them to accomplish chiropractic adjustments. Someone among them transferred the mumps virus to her. The chiropractor's saliva-producing gland, the parotid, lying in the hollow area under and in front of the earlobe, swelled immediately following an extensive dental repair.

"I believe that the mumps had been hanging around in my parotid for a very long time, perhaps for years. I had fevers, chills, headache, weakness, and a general sick feeling beginning a day before the swelling started. I tried all kinds of remedies to treat the symptoms: herbs, homeopathics, chiropractic, and more," Dr. Roberts explained. "Finally, one of my professional colleagues suggested that I take olive leaf extract. I started with one 500-milligram capsule per day and increased the dosage gradually until the inflammation disappeared. Then I went on six capsules a day and eventually elevated the dosage to nine per day for a couple of days. The whole process of healing my mumps took about nine days, which is a short time for an adult." The mumps is considered to be more serious in adults than children, especially for men because the virus can infect a man's testicles.[13]

"I am now using olive leaf extract for my patients; I've dispensed it to them with pleasure. It's awesome in its effect! I'm finding that all of the herpes viruses respond well to it, and I've combined the amino acid lysine with the extract to protect the patient's nerve sheaths. I think that's a good idea,'' said the chiropractor. ''I felt the calcium elenolate in olive leaf was working all through my ear and trigeminal areas, the top and bottom, and up into the forehead. I think the mumps infection had pervaded my body for a number of years and the calcium elenolate got rid of it. Any subclinical infection that I've had lingering in my body must be gone as well, because now I feel perky, uplifted, and full of energy.

''I fully intend remaining on this olive leaf extract for the rest of my life. I can't think of anything better to take as an illness preventative. I anticipate taking two or three capsules a day, along with my other nutritional supplements,'' Dr. Penelope Roberts assured me.

CHAPTER 10

❧

Antibacterial Properties of Olive Leaf Extract

In Willowdale, a suburb of North Toronto, Ontario, Canada, Donald Gay, D.C., HMD, ND, L.Ac., utilizes the olive leaf compound in his combined chiropractic-homeopathic-naturopathic-acupuncture practice. Dr. Gay finds the olive leaf extract especially applicable for the treatment of his patients with chronic fatigue and immune dysfunction syndrome (CFIDS).

"My observation is that CIFIDS patients have an impaired immune ability, leading to assorted infections with viruses and bacteria," Dr. Gay says. "The stress levels in these people adversely alter the functioning of their adrenal glands so that they suffer from absolute adrenal fatigue. This kind of chronic fatigue leads to an elevation in excretion of cortisol, which in turn decreases a person's DHEA [dihydroepiandrosterone] level. Thus the chronic fatigue syndrome patient's immune function further depresses.

"What has been needed for treating this illness is something that rids the person of bacterial, fungal, parasitic, and viral infections, and now I've found the appropriate compound. I see that olive leaf extract does very well for patients suffering from these incidental infections," states Dr. Gay.

"I'm dispensing it in varying amounts, depending on how ill the patient is. Sometimes the quantity of antimicrobial material must be diminished because of the 'die-off' effect it creates [see Chapter 2]. The patient's body occasionally responds with a die-off reaction to the toxins of his or her viruses, bacteria, and other organisms.

"The olive leaf product has been manufactured as liquid, tablets, capsules, powder, and caplets," explains Dr. Gay. "While it's most convenient to use capsules of olive leaf extract, at first I had preferred the powder form. It was my procedure to use the tiny spoon that accompanied this powder. My prescription for patients had been to start with the equivalent of about one-quarter teaspoonful of powder. As I'll mention to you later, I've changed my standard treatment with olive leaf extract and now utilize the capsules.

"Besides chronic fatigue syndrome, I also recommend the extract for use against sore throats, coughs, and chronic sinus problems. I had chronic sinusitis myself—suffered with this bacterial infection of the sinuses for over ten years. Olive leaf extract definitely knocked the long-standing infection out of me within three-and-a-half weeks," says Dr. Gay. "I don't have any more postnasal drip or chronic cough. In all those years of trying every kind of natural or drug remedy—including homeopathics—nothing else worked like this product that's extracted from olives.

"Olive leaf extract acted for me like an herbal antibiotic; it actually killed the sinusitis bacteria. I took one-quarter teaspoonful of powdered extract morning and night. One of the product's manufacturers supplied it to me in the powder form, which I spooned into gelatin capsules. Filling these plain gelatin capsules made it easier for me to take the herbal extract until I changed my procedure. Now I strictly use the finished capsules, which I buy in bottles of sixty because they're so much more convenient," Dr. Donald Gay says.

Sinusitis Often Arises from a Long-standing Bacterial Infection

Dr. Gay's chronic sinusitis may have begun as long ago as decades before, as cold symptoms from a viral infection (see Chapter 9). Because inadequate treatment probably followed then, the lingering condition of sinus obstruction from nasal congestion may have allowed bacteria to invade. Chronic sinusitis often arises from a long-standing bacterial infection.

The repeat symptoms or complications of sinusitis, a relatively superficial, low-grade infection that's uncomfortable but not life-threatening, commonly come back during the same season year after year. The complications occur by extension either through lymphatic channels or by direct involvement of other areas. For example, there may be drainage into the tonsillar area with swelling of the cervicle lymph nodes at the angle of the jaw. There could be infection of the pharynx from the paranasal sinuses through the natural openings. Similarly, the eustachian tube is frequently involved and leads to acute infections of the middle ear (otitis media). Both the sinusitis and the otitis media sometimes develop into chronic, purulent processes.

An estimated 35 million people each year develop sinusitis. According to a recent survey by Yankelovich Partners for the American Academy of Otolaryngology (the organization of physicians performing head and neck surgery), the actual number of affected people may be higher owing to widespread confusion about the signs and symptoms of sinusitis. Most of the bacteria that bring on sinusitis are increasingly resistant to common antibiotics, threatening the efficacy of traditional therapies. The bacteria, *S. pneumoniae* and *H. influenzae,* cause at least 74 percent of all sinusitis cases. *S. aureus* is another bacterium that causes sinusitis. When certain areas of the sinuses are infected, it is considered a medical emergency because of potential damage to

the brain and eyes. Severe headaches usually accompany
these bacterial forms of sinusitis.

Hemolytic Streptococci Cause Sinusitis and Bronchitis, too

Most of the time, such a bacterial sinusitis condition
becomes complicated by the invasion of another biologically
diverse group of microorganisms, identified as the hemolytic
streptococci. They are gram-positive, spherical- or oval-
shaped bacteria that tend to grow in long chains and possess
primary pathogenicity for man and animals. The complicating streptococcus causing chronic sinusitis is a fine example
of how subtle symptoms that return repeatedly make life
miserable for a sufferer.[1]

Such streptococci are one of the sources of acute bacterial
exacerbation of chronic bronchitis, too, a disease that affects
at least 13.8 million Americans. Chronic bronchitis is persistent inflammation of the air passages (bronchi) that connect
the windpipe to the lungs. It's a prolonged, persistent condition with low symptom intensity, occurring when chronic
bronchitis is present on most days for at least three months
per year, for two or more consecutive years. Conditions
associated with chronic bronchitis include:

- Long-term inflammation of the breathing passages
- Enlargement of the mucus glands under the epithelium
  (respiratory tract lining), producing increased amounts
  of mucus
- Impairment of the cilia which line the lungs' mucus
  membranes, complicating mucus discharge
- Upper chest pain, which worsens with a cough

Chronic bronchitis and emphysema often occur together
and typically are the result of cigarette smoking. They are

referred to collectively as chronic obstructive pulmonary disease (COPD). There's reason that COPD is being described here. It's responsive to olive leaf extract. That's because damage to the epithelium from chronic bronchitis predisposes individuals to pneumococcal bacterial invasion, which can lead to further complications, such as pneumonia. Acute exacerbations of chronic bronchitis are identified clinically by two main sets of characteristics:

- Increased cough and labored respiration
- Change in nature and amount of discharges from the respiratory passages

Bacteria that lead to acute bacterial exacerbation of chronic bronchitis include *S. pneumoniae, H. influenzae, M. catarrhalis,* and the hemolytic streptococci. Inasmuch as all of them have already become resistant to traditional antibiotics—these dangerous bacteria don't respond to the usual medical treatment anymore—olive leaf extract is the treatment of choice.

Bacteria as Parasites

A *parasite* is a life form that lives on or in another life form, known as the *host*. *Infection* is parasitism of the host by a microorganism, and *bacterial infection* is a commonly observed form of parasitism of the human host by bacteria.

When parasitism by bacteria results in host injury, the expression of that injury is labeled *bacterial disease*. Bacterial disease is due to *pathogenic* (disease-producing) properties intrinsic to bacteria.

Virulence is the degree of pathogenicity of a bacterial parasite for a host. Different bacteria vary widely in their virulence. Some species of bacteria are highly virulent and cause disease in normal hosts, whereas others are weakly virulent and produce disease only in hosts with deficient defenses against bacterial invasion.[2]

The human host has developed both natural and acquired mechanisms of defense to protect itself from pathogenic bacteria. However, in our overly industrialized environment, with its highly technological setting, sometimes our physiologies can't cope with pathogenic bacteria. We need help from the outside, such as natural antimicrobials or drugs like the antibiotics. In fact, society has allowed medical doctors and osteopathic physicians to overprescribe certain manufactured marvels against bacterial infection, and now we are paying the price with the return of "bad news" bacteria, those antibiotic-resistant, new germ types against which we have no drugs for fending them off.

The "Bad News" Bacteria Now Resistant to Antibiotics

Streptococci, staphylococci, mycobacteria, clostridia, pseudomonas, enterobacteriaceae, spirochetes, salmonella, and the full family of anaerobes are among the vast number of "bad news" bacterial organisms that have become resistant to antibiotics. On the one hand, few therapies rival the success of antibiotics, which have helped cure millions of people of syphilis, pneumonia, tuberculosis, meningitis, gonorrhea, and the myriad of "staph," "strep," and other infections that would otherwise be disabling, if not fatal. However, bacteria have shown amazing ingenuity in developing resistance mechanisms that render potent antibiotics ineffective. The public now faces the same dangers from bacterial infections that were present before the discovery of antibiotics.

With each successive wave of antibiotics produced since the sulfa drugs just before World War II, bacterial organisms have rallied with biochemical self-defenses. Genetic particles conferring resistance to one or several antibiotics have been passed among bacteria by sexual reproduction, and those particles have enabled the germs to become resistant to drugs they had never met.

The problem of resistance has worsened, and the list of better defended organisms has kept growing. Even fifteen years ago, the federal Centers for Disease Control and Prevention in Atlanta reported widespread resistance in the bacterium that causes leprosy to dapsone, the main drug used to treat the disease. This tragedy has led to an elevation in the number of leprosy cases throughout the world.

Among other examples of resistant organisms are bacteria that cause tuberculosis, gonorrhea, cholera, salmonellosis, and pneumonia. Best known, perhaps, is the case of staphylococci which, beginning as long ago as the 1950s, became resistant to penicillin and then to other antibiotics such as methicillin. Infections caused by methicillin-resistant staphylococci hit hard at patients in hospitals, and the problem is continuing even today. The problem is particularly serious in the tertiary care hospitals that treat the most severely ill patients with burns, trauma, cancer, and other disorders. The problem of mutant bacteria has become worldwide. In England and Wales, for instance, over the past twenty-five years, doctors have noted a tenfold increase in urinary tract infections caused by bacteria that are resistant to the antibiotics that once had worked against them.

There undoubtedly had been an overuse of antibiotics in general, which exacerbated the resistance phenomenon among pathological bacteria. Misuse has led to further lessening of antibiotics' effectiveness, loss of lives, and rising costs of treating infections. It turns out that the United States is better off than some countries, where antibiotics are purchased over the counter without prescriptions, leading many people to treat themselves for ailments that do not require antibiotic use.

Still, some North American physicians continue to prescribe antibiotics unnecessarily, as in treatment of viral infections, for which they are ineffective. In the United States and elsewhere, antibiotics are used in feedstuffs to aid the growth of animals for commercial purposes. Consequently, many consumers are overwhelmed with antibacterial substances, ingested in our meat and poultry.

Fortunately, all of us today have the new/old, natural and nontoxic answer for counteracting antibiotic-resistant bacteria, in the form of crystallized calcium elenolate that is present in the oleuropein of olive leaves. This hydrolysized compound of the oleuropein substance is powdered and encapsulated as a food supplement.

Finally, the pressure has been taken off pharmaceutical industry researchers who are no longer coming up with new drugs to intervene in the antibiotic resistance cycle. The American medical consumers have olive leaf extract.

The Antibacterial Attributes of Olive Leaf Extract

Greek bureaucrats in the offices of the Institute of Food Technology at the Ministry of Agriculture in Athens, Greece, have long sought a means of stimulating the fermentative processing of olives (by lactic acid pickling performed by bacteria) as another financial outlet for their country's chief agricultural crop. Still, because of the well-characterized oleuropein component in the olive tree, the antibacterial effect is so strong it must be removed before any fermentation can take place. Olive oil fermentation is caused by those specific lactic acid bacteria which release enzymes to produce a chemical change in the olives.[3]

At least six major phenolic components of extracts from green olives and their leaves have been associated with the inhibition of the two major advantageously fermentative bacterial organisms, *Lactobacillus plantarum* and *Leuconostoc mesenteroides*.[4] Until approximately 1970, the olive fermentation industry had suffered severe financial losses from the antibiotic peculiarity of their crop, but then an agricultural advancement gave olive tree growers the way out of their dilemma.

Waste Waters from Olive Washing May Become a New Industry

As mentioned above, the waste waters derived from the milling of olive paste during olive oil production are richly antibiotic. The olive paste manufacturing process is accompanied by continuous washing with water, a procedure I have referred to in an earlier chapter as *malaxation*. The resulting water was discarded by the olive oil industry as a waste product until the new olive leaf extract was developed.[5] As the result of revelations explained in this book, an entirely new industry may now be arising which uses olive washing waste water as an antimicrobial by-product.

In the event such waste waters find their way into the soil, the presence of the olive tree's antimicrobial substances adversely affect biodegradation. They displace beneficial soil members of the bacterial flora which are susceptible.[6] These soil members especially include aerobic spore-forming bacteria.[7] In a recent study, Dr. Jose M. Rodriguez and his coworkers in Athens, Greece, and Valencia, Spain, who worked with *Bacillus megaterium,* found that waste waters from olive processing mills inhibited growth of vegetative cells as well as the processes of germination and sporulation.[8]

As mentioned, the discovery of how to make an olive extract using "waste waters" from olive oil production may have brought forth this whole new industry in antibiotic/antiviral/antifungal/antiprotozoan agent production. This will be a benefit not only for the growers of olive trees but also for those multimillions of people who must attempt to cope with devastating microbial infections—most especially the invasion of bacteria and other disease-producing microorganisms.

More investigations have been conducted, and they show

that extracts taken from olive leaves inhibit microfungi and pathogenic bacteria.[9] The protein secretions of *Staphylococcus aureus* cease when it comes into the proximity of olive leaf extract.[10] Thus, "staph" infections are now controllable, and even eradicatable, without the need for antibiotics because of this newfound olive leaf extract.

Table 7 presents a list of bacteria and other dangerous germs inhibited or killed by olive leaf extract in laboratory tests conducted by The Upjohn Company. The herbal substance has been proven by Upjohn to be virucidal, bactericidal, fungicidal, candidicidal, and parasiticidal. The recently discovered phytochemicals in olive leaves, taken as a supplement to the diet, have undergone toxicity testing as well, and produced no adverse side effects in laboratory animals.[11]

The Very Serious Bacillus cereus Infection

Someone who becomes infected with a truly debilitating bacterial organism, *Bacillus cereus*, is struck by repeated cycles of nausea; belching; indigestion; copious gas; frothing spittle or vomit; frothy diarrhea; burning stomach, requiring massive amounts of antacids; sore abdomen; muscular weakness and pain in the upper arms, neck, chest, and just above the knee; plus extreme fatigue with the least movement.

In addition, there are heart symptoms with *B. cereus* contamination: heart rate fluctuation from 34 to 160 beats per minute; electrocardiogram readings showing changes similar to those seen in diphtheria and other bacterial toxins; and possible permanent nerve damage to the heart. Also the *B. cereus* infection brings on bone pain so severe a victim can't sit or lie in one position for prolonged periods without feeling a deep ache in the bones. There are temperature changes in the body going from severe chills to excessive sweating.

The *B. cereus* patient additionally undergoes mental con-

TABLE 7

An *In Vitro* Paper Disk Bioassay Conducted by The Upjohn Company Indicates That Olive Leaf Extract Is Effective Against a Minimum of Fifty-Six (56) Disease-Causing Organisms, Including the Following Bacteria, Viruses, Fungi, Yeasts and Protozoa:

(Accompanying numbers, names, and letters identify the species' strain)

Herpes	Reovirus (Deering)
Vaccinia	Maloney murine leukemia
Pseudorabies	Rauscher murine leukemia
Influenza A (PRS)	Moloney sarcoma
Newcastle disease	Influenza A/NWS (HONI)
Parainfluenza 3	In. A/PR8/34 (HONI)
Coxsackie A 21	In. A/FM/1/47 (HONI)
Encephalomyocarditis	In. A/Ann Arbor/1/57 (HIN2)
Polio 1	In. A/Hong Kong/Richardson/68 (H3N2)
Polio 2	In. B/Lee/40
Polio 3	In. B/Maryland/1/59
Vesicular Stomititus	Lactobacillus plantarum (W50)
Sindbis	L. brevis 50
Parainfluenza 1 (Sendai) ATCC	Pediococcus cerevisiac 39
Para. 1 (Sendai) TUC	Leuconostoc mesenteroides 42
Para. 1 (C-35, HA-2)	Staphylococcus aureus
Para. 2 (CA, Greer)	Bacillus subtilis
Enterobacteraerogenes NRRL B-199	E. cloacae NRRL B-414
Escherichia coli	Salmonella typhimurium
Pseudomonas fluorescens	Erwinia carotovora
P. Solanacearum	E. tracheiphila
P. lachrymans	Xanthomonas vesicatoria
Corynebacterium michiganese	Plasmodium falciparum
Virax	Malariac

Pediococcus cerevisiae 39	Saccharomyces rosei NRRL Y-1567
Kloeckera apiculata NRRL Y-1380	Candida krusei NRRL Y-105
S. cerevisiae var. ellipsoideus NRRL Y-635	Hansenula subpelliculosa NRRL Y-1455
Debaryomyces membranaefaciens NRRL Y-1455	Pichia membranaefaciens NRRL Y-1627

fusion, extreme depression, loss of the will to live, plus abdominal distension and pain. Complicating all the other troubles are respiratory inflammation and permanent lung damage. The inability to absorb food and resultant weight loss gradually come upon the individual. Finally death ensues. There has been no known effective treatment for *Bacillus cereus* infection, and surely not any cure.[12]

The Newly Discovered Cure for Bacillus cereus

Bacillus cereus is an aerobic, rod-shaped, gram-positive (spore-forming) bacterium. This pathogen is ubiquitous in human and animal environments. It is frequently present in small numbers in common foods such as potatoes, carrots, and celery. Sometimes, the bacillus is responsible for food poisoning arising from eating fried rice in a Chinese restaurant, when the rice has sat overnight in a wok and been reheated the next day. Know the kitchen status of the restaurant which you patronize; otherwise, the individual who loves to eat fried rice could be in danger of coming down with an infection of *B. cereus*. The incubation period for gastrointestinal symptoms range from one to six hours and, in usual cases, last for less then twenty-four hours.[13]

B. cereus processes an enterotoxin, which activates the intestinal enzyme adenylate cyclase (an isomeric nucleotide). This enzymatic action results in intestinal fluid secretion. Thus two contrasting forms of illness may result: first, vomiting (emetic) illness with the triple upper-gastrointestinal-tract symptoms of nausea, vomiting, and flatulence (rather like staphylococcal food poisoning), and second, diarrheal illness with lower-intestinal-tract symptoms involving the production of diarrhea and rectal gas (much as in *Clostridium perfringens* food poisoning).

The diagnosis cannot be confirmed in patients by isolation of *B. cereus* from their stools unless negative stool cultures are obtained from a suitable control group of patients. Although *B. cereus* grows readily on a nonselective medium, such as plain agar or blood agar, most bacteriology laboratories will not look for the organism unless identification is specifically requested by the attending physician.[14]

Today there is good treatment and possibly a cure for *B. cereus.* The newly discovered phenolic compounds extracted from olives and their leaves with ethyl acetate inhibits germination (reproduction) and outgrowth of *Bacillus cereus* T spores. Purified oleuropein present in olive leaves, but modified by a manufacturing process so that it becomes activated in the olive leaf extract, inhibits the germination and growth process of the infecting bacterium.

A 1991 laboratory study on phenolic compounds and oleuropein made some significant observations related to victims of *B. cereus* infections. The addition of oleuropein and olive leaf extract either (1) to the *in vitro* growth of *B. cereus,* or (2) to a prophylactic/therapeutic nutritional supplementation regimen for patients within three to five minutes after germination of the organism begins, immediately decreases the rate of change for *B. cereus* from phase bright to phase dark spores. This color change noted under the microscope shows that the pathological microbe is being altered to the point of death, or at least to growth inhibition. Olive leaf extract taken as a food supplement delays significant outgrowth of the pathogen.[15]

Researchers at the Athens Institute of Food Technology

who were the authors of the above-cited study of *B. cereus* T spores wrote: "... the addition of oleuropein and olive leaf extract at various times during the process of germination inhibit the outgrowth of the germinated spores." Twenty-three years before, other Greek scientists concluded that inhibition takes place from denaturation of germination enzymes by means of inhibition of the lytic enzyme subtilopeptidase A.[16] In addition, researchers suggest that there is interference with the bacterium's use of the amino acid L-alanine or other amino acids necessary for the initiation of its germination process.[17]

More Information About Oleuropein

During interviews for articles and this book on olive leaf extract, California clinician James Privitera, M.D., told me that numerous researchers throughout Europe have found "... that oleuropein inactivates bacteria by dissolving the outer lining of the microbes. Another team of scientists determined that oleuropein, and specifically its elenolic acid component, inhibits the growth of certain species of lactic acid bacteria used in the brining [salting] and fermenting of olives."

From what's been read to this point, you know that the chemical substance, oleuropein, is the compound responsible for the disease-resistant properties long known to be present in the olive tree's fruit, bark, root, and leaf.[18] Oleuropein can be hydrolyzed by mineral acids, changing its glucosidic and ester bonds. The intermediate compound formed by such a hydrolyzing action spontaneously rearranges the altered oleuropein into a new virucidal, bacterocidal, fungicidal, and parasiticidal compound that was identified by Upjohn Company biochemists and other researchers in the olive oil industry as (-)-elenolic acid.[19] There is no question that, *in vitro,* it possesses all these antimicrobial characteristics.[20] To a limited extent, the (-)-elenolic acid also works the same way *in vivo.*[21]

In 1934 and 1935 it was demonstrated that the action of beta-glucosidase, the olive leaf's enzyme, on oleuropein was such that it produces a product which turns spectral light shining through its crystals to the right (dextrorotary).[22] In addition, there is another olive tree enzyme with the formula (+)-2-epielenolic acid present in the olive fruit which cleaves the ester linkages of oleuropein.[23]

Olive leaf extract exerts its main influence by *in vivo* hydrolysis of oleuropein to (+)-2-epielenolic acid. The way this chemical hydrolysis gets accomplished is suspected by chemists to take place through the action of serum beta-glucosidase and serum esterase.

Olive Leaf Extract Treatment for Other Bacterial Infections

Speaking of clinical responses to the product, Dr. Privitera advised, "One of my patients with a painful abscessed tooth took several olive leaf extract capsules at night to reduce the pain so he could sleep. It worked, and he slept well. The next morning some pain and swelling had returned; therefore, he then took a 'handful' of them again—about eight or nine of the capsules. An hour-and-a-half later the pain and swelling were gone. The infection and pain never returned, although the tooth eventually became loose, gradually blackened, and was extracted."

Naturopath Philip Selinsky, N.D., at the Institute for Holistic Studies in Santa Barbara, California, states: "Sinus and bladder infections caused by bacteria have responded well to olive leaf extract along with oral infections associated with mucous membrane infections and with tooth or gum disease. They have been particularly responsive. Some patients have told me that the olive leaf extract capsules I dispensed to them took down their dental-related infections in a matter of hours. The response is quite impressive."

For bacterial infections of the teeth and the bladder too,

Dr. Selinsky recommends that patients should start with two olive leaf extract capsules followed by another one every four hours—about eight to ten in a day is the correct dose. "That dosage usually gets you on top of the dental or bladder infection situation," he says. "For more serious infections, the capsules can be taken at shorter intervals."

America still has a long way to go in preventing the spread of contagious diseases, if data from the National Notifiable Diseases Surveillance System (NNDSS) is any indication. The surveillance system tracks fifty-two infectious diseases in the United States each year. Of the ten most frequently reported illnesses, 87 percent of all cases were sexually transmitted. The United States has the highest rate of sexually transmitted diseases of any developed country. The University of Texas, Houston Health Science Center, advises that the ten most frequently reported infectious diseases in 1995, as shown in Table 8 (in their descending order of frequency), are:

TABLE 8

America's Top Ten Reported Infectious Diseases of 1995

1. Chlamydia
2. Gonorrhea
3. AIDS
4. Salmonellosis
5. Hepatitis A
6. Shigellosis
7. Tuberculosis
8. Primary and Secondary Syphilis
9. Lyme Disease
10. Hepatitis B

Source: "Top ten reported infectious diseases of 1995." *UT Lifetime Health Letter*, The University of Texas, Houston Health Science Center, Vol. 9, No. 1, Jan. 1997, p. 2.

❧

CHAPTER 11

Correction for the Yeast Syndrome and Other Fungal Diseases

From his cabin in a wilderness area located about three hours by car north of Sacramento, California, Michael Rothback, D.Sc., Ph.D., a thirty-eight-year-old assistant professor in physics at the University of California, telephoned me about having suffered from the yeast syndrome. Dr. Rothback had his condition for four years before finally ridding himself of it by using olive leaf extract. The corrective remedy had been suggested as good treatment for generally boosting his immune system by licensed acupuncturist Frank Campanale, LAc., of Redding, California, a member of the California State Board of Acupuncture Orthopedics.

"A lot of my patient therapy consists of Chinese herbal medicine and homeopathy," explained Mr. Campanale. "Olive leaf extract being an herbal therapy, I have a dozen people taking it, and some are doing quite well. Those with the yeast syndrome or other common fungal conditions have an especially good result from using olive leaf extract. It works against fungus infection of the nails, athlete's foot, jock itch, tinea capitis, and other fungal diseases. But the yeast syndrome is where olive leaf extract is most effective in my hands."

The yeast syndrome is a systemic fungal infection identified by wholistic health professionals as *candidiasis,* which actually begins in the gut and spreads to other areas of the body. Fungi are somewhat common invaders of the body which produce disease symptoms and signs. A great variety of drug therapies are employed as treatment, but none are very effective; otherwise, there would not be the need for so many of them.

Common Fungal Foes That Cause Disease

Fungi are filamentous, parasitic plants consisting of single-cell life forms which inhabit the land, air, and waters of the earth. They belong to that part of the vegetable kingdom known as *Thallophytes,* which exist everywhere. They reproduce by budding or making spores, and are more highly developed than the viruses and bacteria. The fungi obtain their food from organic matter, synthesized by other organisms; thereby, they differ from algae, which also belong to the Thallophytes. The algae have chlorophyl and are able to obtain food from inorganic compounds by their own synthetic means, aided by the energy of sunlight. As noted, fungi don't do that and vary from the higher plant forms by growing in irregular masses, not differentiated into roots, stems, and leaves.[1]

It's estimated by mycologists, scientists who study fungi as their specialty, that over half-a-million different fungal species inhabit the earth. Yeasts are fungi. Some fungi are edible, such as the mushrooms, but thirty others are foes of humankind. At least eight primary classifications of fungal families cause disease processes: the dermatomycoses, candidiasis, maduromycosis, sporotrichosis, blastomycosis, actinomycosis, coccidiodides, torulosis, and aspergillosis. The dermatomycoses and candidiasis affect North Americans and Europeans. The others cause troubles for people living in more tropical settings, such as Australia, Equatorial

Africa, Southern Asia, the Pacific Rim, Central America, and the Amazonian area of South America.

The fungi are survivalists, changing their form from rapid growth to no growth, and can remain that way for thousands of years, such as those found as living spores in Egyptian tombs. Fungi make poisons called mycotoxins which produce discomforting symptoms of disease in all populations, but especially in those of the industrialized countries.

If plants, animals, and humans stay alive and well in a state of homeostasis, the fungi that exist all around them are unable to overcome the immunity mechanisms which these higher forms of life possess. Their natural defenses often interfere with fungal actions. But once death overtakes the living animal or plant, these fungi are the principal undertakers and managers; they reduce all that have ever lived on earth into the molecules from which they were assembled. In science, biochemists refer to this reductionist function of fungi as "the carbon cycle," while philosophers may describe their natural actions as "coming from dust and going to dust."

Of course, there is one exception to this simple balanced equation of life and death, which is that the fungi can attack living plants and animals while they are alive as well. For instance, a person might contract a non-life-threatening fungal infection between the toes (athlete's foot) which could be easily eradicated with some topical over-the-counter remedy. At the opposite extreme is the patient with a compromised immune system which has lost its effectiveness against opportunistic fungi. This immune-suppressed individual will be likely to face a variety of death-dealing major fungal infections, as occurs in AIDS, and require all kinds of prescription drugs. In between these extremes are ongoing fungal infections associated with chronic diseases such as diabetes, cancer, and other degenerative conditions, including cross infections as with the yeast overgrowth of *Candida albicans* that lodges inside the gut.

Many fungal (mycotic) infections of various anatomical

parts, within the body and on the skin surface, are adversely affected by the antifungal effects of olive leaf extract. Table 9 offers a listing that ranges from bacteria-like fungi to yeast or yeast-like organisms, against which olive leaf extract may show efficacy. Sometimes a variety of names have been given by mycologists to the same species. As a result, although mycology is older than the study of bacteriology, it has lagged far behind in its classification and practical application of general knowledge. Such a state of affairs for mycology should now change, because olive leaf extract may prove itself effective against all fungi, including yeasts, algae, and molds.

TABLE 9

The Classification of Fungi Against Which Olive Leaf Extract May Be Fungicidal or Fungistatic [2]

(Listed are the fungi most frequently encountered in human infections.)

I. ALGAE (containing chlorophyl)
II. FUNGI (containing no chlorophyl)
   A. SCHIZOMYCETES (bacteria)
      1. *Actinomycetaceae*
         a. *Actinomyces israeli (bovis) (anaerobic or micro-aerophilic)*
         b. *Nocardia* (obligate aerobic)
            (1) *asteroides*
            (2) *madurae*
            (3) *tenius*
            (4) *minutissima*
   B. MYXOMYCETES (slime molds)
   C. EUMYCETES (true fungi)
      1. PHYCOMYCETES (mycelium nonseptate)
         a. *Mucor* sp. and *Rhizopus* sp.
      2. BASIDIOMYCETES (mycelium septate, sexual spores exogenous)
      3. ASCOMYCETES (mycelium septate, sexual spores endogenous)

4. FUNGI IMPERFECTI (no sexual spores)
   a. *Cryptococcus neoformans*
   b. *Candida albicans*
   c. *Geotrichum* sp.
   d. *Blastomyces dermatitidis*
   e. *Blastomyces brasiliensis*
   f. *Histoplasma capsulatum*
   g. *Sporotrichum schenckii*
   h. *Coccidiodes immitis*
   i. *Aspergillus* sp.
   j. *Pencillium* sp.
   k. *Hormodendrum (cladosprium)*
      (1) *pedrosoi*
      (2) *compactum*
      (3) *tricoides*
      (4) *wernecki*
   l. *Phialophora verrucosa*
   m. *Microsporum*
      (1) *audouini*
      (2) *canis*
      (3) *gypseum*
   n. *Epidermophyton floccosum*
   o. *Trichophyton*
      (1) *mentagrophytes*
      (2) *rubrum*
      (3) *tonsurans*
      (4) *epilans*
      (5) *sabouraudi*
      (6) *sulfureum*
      (7) *schoenleini*
      (8) *concentricum*
      (9) *ferrugineum*
      (10) *violaceum*
      (11) *faviforme*
   p. *Rhinosporidum*
   q. *Malassezia furfur*
   r. *Piedraia hortai*
   s. *Trichosporon beigelii*

Source: See Chapter 11, reference 2, in the References at the back of the book.

The Yeast Syndrome Present in All of Us

Of the numerous pathological fungal organisms infecting people who live in industrialized countries, the one most often producing disease symptoms comes from a species of yeast. The yeast syndrome is a harmful infection caused by the fungus *Candida albicans,* the predominant commensal yeast present in all of us. Most often it resides in a saprophytic (neutral) fashion and remains harmless. However, sometimes it turns ugly.

Toxins produced by this pathogenic/parasitic form of fungus get absorbed into the body and cause devastating symptoms. Chronic fatigue is its predominant manifestion as it overgrows in the gut, the vagina, the mouth, several internal organs, and some other body regions. Conditions associated with the yeast syndrome include acne, allergies, anxiety, asthma, constipation, depression, diarrhea, earaches, headaches, infertility, lost sex drive, poor memory, muscle weakness, persistent coughs, premenstrual syndrome, recurrent vaginitis, skin irritations, and dozens more.

The yeast syndrome's host—almost any human being in which, or on which, this fungus lives—sometimes experiences symptoms when colonies of the infecting species start to grow and spread around the body. The yeast is normally controlled by your body's immune defenses and by the usual friendly bacterial flora present in it. But when a sudden or gradual ecological change takes place in the internal environment, helpful bacteria tend to decrease and immune response becomes depressed. Then, since the yeast is an "opportunistic organism," it begins to increase in the body, especially in one's colon.

Alan S. Levin, M.D., Adjunct Professor of Immunology in the Department of Dermatology, University of California, San Francisco, explains: "*Candida albicans* is an opportunistic organism. If a circumstance occurs in your body to upset the delicate intestinal balance, such an opportunistic organism will strive to gain a firmer hold and colonize throughout the human gut and possibly other tissues. Intestinal imbalance with subsequent immune suppression occurs from the taking of antibiotics, eating excessive amounts of simple carbohydrates, consuming yeasty foods, engaging in sexual promiscuity, taking street drugs, and/or following a generally unhealthy lifestyle.''[3]

General Characteristics of the Yeast Syndrome

Invading yeast colonies do their damage by releasing powerful chemicals, toxins characteristic of the Candida organism. Hence the poisons are called *canditoxins,* which may be absorbed into the bloodstream, causing widely diverse symptoms. In addition to adults, yeast affects children, too, giving them diaper rash, thrush, and possibly some really serious disease manifestations such as autism and minimal brain dysfunction.

The yeast syndrome is officially known to wholistic and biological physicians by the scientific term *polysystemic chronic candidiasis.* However, allopathic physicians who practice conventionally may still not acknowledge the existence of the yeast syndrome. When these uneducated or narrow-minded doctors are forced to refer to this chronic, generalized disease entity (which at one time or other has affected 34 percent of the population on earth), they usually call the condition *candidiasis hypersensitivity syndrome.*

Sixty years ago doctors identified *Candida albicans* as a frequent cause of vagina, mouth, throat, and gastrointestinal tract infections. Now it's well known to invade almost all body parts, organs, tissues, and cells. The organism is believed to be a complicating factor in severe pathological conditions. For instance, research physicians suspect the Candida family as a complication in acquired immune deficiency syndrome (AIDS), a contributor to early death in various forms of cancer (especially leukemia), a source of infertility in some women, and a mischief-maker in other medical tragedies such as multiple sclerosis, myasthenia gravis, disseminated lupus erythematosis, schizophrenia, arthritis, and many other degenerative diseases.

How the Organism Changes from Neutral to Pathological

Ordinarily *Candida albicans* is a commensal organism with humans and other animals as its host. *Commensal* means that it lives in and on the host without either harming or benefiting them. For example, Candida lives in our intestines, the gut, obtaining both food and suitable habitat but not affecting us in any way. Normally it is also a saprophyte— a germ that lives by eating dead tissue rather than living matter. But when you undergo ecological change within your body from too much enjoyment of our society's high-tech lifestyles and your immune system finally succumbs to unnatural living, *Candida albicans* changes also.

It loses its commensal and saprophytic characteristics. From being a commensal organism, Candida changes into a parasite. From a saprophyte, it turns into a pathogen. The yeast, no longer neutral and harmless, now not only contributes nothing to your welfare, but produces irritation, interferes with bodily functions, destroys cells, disrupts organs, damages tissues, and releases canditoxins. Thus it causes disease, promotes injury, deteriorates the quality of life, and potentially brings on early death.

Of its canditoxins, a minimum of seventy-nine known chemical substances exist against which the human body creates an identifiable antibody. Each Candida strain—*C. albicans* being just one among eighty-one strains—has about thirty-five antigens, implying that millions of antigens are possible. Antigens are potentially dangerous foreign substances in the body against which you produce antibodies.

When too much pathogenic yeast has colonized your tissues, the antibodies produced become insufficient to ward off the disease symptoms.

The yeast syndrome can be a very serious condition, probably affecting every third person in the industrialized Western world, and it's expected to affect more. Often it comes on you through no fault of your own. As mentioned, Candida is stimulated to spread by the unnatural effects of high technology, though many people are unaware that technology is a cause of the breaking down of one's immune defenses.

Reasons for the Yeast to Become a Pathogen

When you consume quantities of animal protein like steaks, chops, and other red meats which are loaded with antibiotics, or when you are prescribed broad spectrum antibiotics for the treatment of bacterial infections, these newly introduced drugs tend to turn the Candida saprophyte into a pathogen. Pathogens thrive on living tissue in the human body and are capable of causing infection or disease.

Taking cortisone, birth control pills, or other steriod derivatives creates hormonal imbalance. More than that, the steroids in these products are actually food for the yeast organism. *Candida albicans* grows fat, buds, and gives birth to Candida daughters, which steadily increase their total area of tissue invasion after being converted to pathogen status. They find nourishment in and around your cells.

Aspects of unnatural lifestyles include not only antibiotics and oral contraceptives, but also therapeutic hormones such as estrogen replacement therapy, anti-inflammatory drugs, recreational drugs, foods high in mold or yeast content such as cake, bread, beer, mushrooms, and brewer's yeast, plus a diet with excess refined sugar or the simple carbohydrates contained in junk food.

Something to be aware of is that the average American consumes more than fifty-two teaspoonsful of sugar a day, with 70 percent of it hidden in processed foods such as ketchup, salad dressing, chips, cake mixes, ice cream, and other packaged foods of all types. As it happens, many people in the United States are quite aware of the damage sugar causes within the body's tissues and hardly ingest any sugary products at all. That means that some uninformed Americans take in even larger quantities of the sweet and deadly product. Since simple carbohydrates (sugars) are a main food on which *Candida albicans* thrives, it's no wonder that the yeast syndrome is so rampant among populations in the United States, Canada, England, the Netherlands, France, Germany, and other industrialized countries of the West.

How to Determine Whether the Yeast Syndrome Is Your Problem

How might you determine whether the yeast syndrome is your health problem? Of course, laboratory tests have been developed. Your wholistic physician, naturopath, chiropractor, or another health professional, involved with alternative methods of healing (usually not any doctor who practices conventional AMA-type medicine) is the individual to consult for diagnosis and treatment of the yeast syndrome. Other than visiting your doctor, you can make your own determination in part.

Table 10 gives a partial listing of illnesses which are closely connected to the yeast syndrome. With *C. albicans* infesting the internal and external body parts of everyone, invariably the presence of a few of the following symptoms or conditions indicates that the yeast syndrome is a potential problem for you.

Rather than clinical examinations or laboratory tests, the patient's history and symptoms are usually the keys to making a diagnosis of the yeast syndrome. Chronic symptoms

TABLE **10**

Symptoms, Signs, and Conditions of Illness Proven to be Connected with the Yeast Syndrome

Check yourself against this listing and see if you are affected by any of these difficulties related to chronic, generalized candidiasis, otherwise known as the yeast syndrome.

Agitation	Infections—bacterial, viral, fungal
Allergies	Insomnia—chronic or sudden sporadic
Asthma	Loss of concentration
Body aches	Loss of libido
Chemical sensitivities	Loss of memory
Chronic heartburn	Menstrual irregularities
Chronic infections	Premenstrual anxiety/tension
Colitis	Premenstrual depression/moodiness
Constipation	Sensitivity to odors, chemicals, smoke
Cramping in the belly	Stomach distension/bloating
Depression	Swelling/fluid retention or loading
Diarrhea	Vaginal yeast infection
Disturbed senses: taste, smell, vision, hearing	Weight changes: gain or loss
Dizziness	
	Serious degenerative diseases such as MS, AIDS, ALS, lupus erythematosis, heart disease, Crohn's
Earaches	disease, Hashimoto's disease, endocrine gland dysfunction, diabetes, hepatitis, alopecia, vitiligo,
Gastritis	ovaritis, Addison's disease, myasthenia gravis, pemphigus, schizophrenia, allergic rhinitis, autism,

Headaches	sprue, celiac disease, testiculitis, rheumatoid arthritis, Sjogren's syndrome
Hives	
Hyperactivity (in children)	
Hyperirritability	
Impotence	

I have listed together with a history of using oral contraceptives, steroids, and antibiotics all point to a Candida infection being present. Your lifestyle usually decides if you're a candidate for candidiasis. A lifestyle survey for the yeast syndrome, answered by the patient and taken by a doctor oriented to candidiasis as a clinical entity, is probably the best diagnositic aid. Such a survey is provided following Table 10.

A Lifestyle Survey to Determine If You Have the Yeast Syndrome[4]

There are four parts to the following survey of symptoms and the lifestyle which may be causing them: (A) for adults and teenagers in general, (B) for women only, (C) for men only, and the final one, (D) for children under age ten. The questions for the respective group should be answered "yes" or "no" and the positive responses counted for scoring. Scores of 65 percent or greater (more than three positive responses for questionnaires (A), (B), and (C) may indicate that the yeast syndrome is a causative factor for the presence of symptoms and signs of the yeast syndrome. For questionnaire (D), a score of 75 percent or less (any positive response) is an indication that a child could have the yeast syndrome. Naturally, the higher the score for any of the questionnaires, the more certain it is that discomforts are caused by *Candida albicans*.

A. Questions for Adults and Teenagers

Have you suffered from:

1. Frequent infections, constant skin problems, or taken antibiotics, birth control pills, or cortisone medications often or for long periods?
2. Feelings of fatigue, being drained, drowsiness, or illness symptoms on damp muggy days or in moldy places such as a basement?
3. Feelings of anxiety, irritability, insominia, or cravings for sugary foods, breads, alcoholic beverages?
4. Food sensitivities, allergy reactions, or digestion problems, bloating, heartburn, constipation, bad breath?
5. Feeling "spacey" or "unreal," difficult to concentrate, or bothered by perfumes, chemical fumes, tobacco smoke?
6. Poor coordination, muscle weakness, or joints painful or swollen?
7. Mood swings, depression, or loss of sexual feelings?
8. Dry mouth or throat, nose congestion or drainage, a feeling of pressure above the ears, or frequent headaches?
9. Pains in the chest, shortness of breath, dizziness, or easy bruising?
10. Frustration of going from doctor to doctor, never getting your health completely well, or being told that your symptoms are "mental" or "psychological" or "psychosomatic"?

B. Questions for Women Only

Have you suffered from:

1. Vaginal burning or itching, discharge, infections, or urinary problems?
2. Difficulty getting pregnant?

3. Been pregnant two or more times?
4. Taken birth control pills?
5. Premenstrual symptoms such as moodiness, fluid loading, tension?
6. Irregular menstrual cycles or other menstrual problems?
7. Permanently appearing changes in the time or frequency of menstruation?
8. Heavy discharge from your nipples?
9. Pain during sexual intercourse?
10. Vaginal spotting?
11. Pelvic pain?
12. Breast lumps?
13. Hot flashes?

C. Questions for Men Only

Have you suffered from:

1. Difficulty having an erection?
2. A lump in the testicles?
3. A sore on the penis?
4. Any discharge from the penis?
5. A breast lump?
6. Impotence or premature ejaculation?
7. Peyronie's disease?
8. Loss of libido?
9. Prostatitis?
10. Orchitis (testiculiti)?
11. Pain in the lower abdomen?

D. Questions Especially for Children Under Age Ten

Has the child suffered from:

1. Frequent infections: particularly of the ears, tonsilitis, bronchitis, history of constant diaper rash?
2. Continuous nasal congestion or drainage?

3. Dark circles under the eyes, or periods of hyperactivity, poor attention span?
4. A long history of bedwetting?
5. Eczema?

The four sets of questions above allow you to decide if the yeast syndrome is one of the sets of symptoms and signs contributing to your or a family member's overall discomfiture. Too many positive responses may lead you or your loved one to seek treatment because the high score acknowledges that this uncomfortable body has been invaded by *Candia albicans.* The yeast syndrome is one of the most frequent factors contributing to chronic fatigue and allied symptoms. Keep track of your scoring. As you get better, your scoring will go down.

If you had four or five "yes" answers, you possibly suffer with a yeast-related illness; if you had six or seven "yes" answers, you are probably a Candida infection victim; if you had eight or more "yes" answers, you almost certainly need to get treatment for chronic, generalized candidiasis.

Today's Treatment for Yeast and Other Fungal Diseases

What do we know now, as we approach the beginning of the twenty-first century, that Orion Truss, M.D., the discoverer of the yeast syndrome (systemic candidiasis), did not know in the early 1980s?

A. The usual anticandida pharmaceutical, nystatin, can't completely rid the body of *Candida albicans,* for this drug eventually causes mutation of the candida species into other fungi with subsequent development of nystatin-resistant forms. Furthermore, nystatin does not penetrate the blood/brain barrier to affect mental derangements connected with the disease (schizophrenia is one of its unpleasant effects).

B. More than 30 percent of patients being treated for candida-related complex show problems in maintaining a normal body temperature. According to some scientists, one of the physiological mediators, known as *interleukin-1,* stimulates the immune cells to combat the yeast infection simultaneously with sending a signal to the hypothalamus to increase the body temperature in order to provide an ideal microclimate for the proliferation of the immune cells.

C. It has been found that there is a strong yeast-parasite connection. In his quest to unravel the candida enigma, Warren M. Levin, M.D., of New York City, was the first complementary medicine physician to recognize that parasites and candidiasis usually are present together as pathological entities. In another instance, parasitologist Hermann Bueno, M.D., of New York City and Brooklyn, New York, discovered and implemented a new method for collecting stool specimens containing yeast and parasites, which he named *anoscopy.*

D. Anti-allergy injections containing candida antigens, coupled with anti-fungal treatment and the yeast-free diet, achieve good results against candida-related complex; but there is a decreasing efficacy with this treatment program. That's because of a cross-reactivity between the candida yeast organism, various other yeasts, and the numerous molds. Injecting with a combination of yeasts, molds, and allergens gives better results.

A specific singular treatment has been needed for the yeast syndrome, and finally it has been found. Olive leaf extract is applicable to chronic, systemic candidiasis. It is more potent as treatment than even nystatin or taheebo tea and other commonly used drug and natural remedies.

The Surefire Natural Treatment Program for Candidiasis

When six capsules daily of olive leaf extract, taken in three divided doses, are combined with the natural treatment program established back in 1986 when my coauthored book, *The Yeast Syndrome,* was first published, you will be using a surefire correction method for getting rid of candidiasis.[5] Here is the full program as currently recommended by Pavel Yutsis, M.D., in *The Downhill Syndrome: If Nothing's Wrong, Why Do I feel So Bad?*[6]

- Avoid antibiotic usage unless absolutely mandatory.
- Discontinue birth control pills in the presence of vaginal discharge.
- Apply homeopathic dilutions of candida.
- Consume two fresh garlic cloves daily or substitute aged garlic extract acquired from the health food store.
- Take allergy injections that include antigens containing Tricophyton-Candida-Epidermophyton (TCE) combined with different molds.
- Avoid immune system–suppressing drugs such as steroids, hormones, and anti-inflammatory agents.
- Drink Pau d' arco (also called taheebo or La Pacho) tea.
- Take nutritional supplements each day including 1,200 mg of calcium, 1,200 mg of magnesium, 60 mg of zinc, 4,000 mg of vitamin C, 400 mcg of chromium polynicotinate, 100 mg of B complex, and 15,000 IU of beta-carotene.
- Supplement your diet with those friendly bacteria found in the gut naturally, which aid digestion and fight off the yeast, *Candida albicans.* These advantageous bacteria are known as *probiotics,* and may be acquired from almost any health food store. They should be taken orally in the equivalent of 1.5 billion live beneficial

organisms for each capsule of olive leaf extract used as part of the overall treatment program. The most useful probiotics consist of *Lactobacillus acidophilus, Bifidobacterium bifidum, Lactobacillus bulgaricus, Streptococcus faecium, Bifidobacterium longum,* and other live cultures to restore the body balance.

- At least every other day, eat plenty of plain, unsweetened, nonfruited yogurt made at home or from commercial manufacturers containing similar live cultures of beneficial bacteria as mentioned above.

- Ingest naturally occurring short-chain fatty acids such as caprylic acid as nutritional supplementation.

- Eat a natural anti-yeast diet, such as the one utilized by Dr. Yutsis. He refers to it as the FAVER diet, consisting of Fish, All meats that are antibiotic-free, Vegetables, Eggs, and Rice cakes.

- As part of the FAVER diet, don't expose yourself to any yeast foods that provide nourishment for the stimulation of yeast growth. For a full description of edibles to consume and not to consume when you are affected by an overgrowth of *Candida albicans,* see the extensive tables and alphabetical listings of foods shown on pages 196 through 246 in *The Yeast Syndrome.* That reference guide remains the dietary foundation which almost all wholistic physicians who treat candidiasis use as the basis for their patients' food preparation, daily menus, recipes, and other parts of the eating program.

CHAPTER 12

❦

How to Expel the Parasites Living Within Us

In private practice as a licensed acupuncturist in Santa Monica, California, doctor of oriental medicine Timothy Ray, O.M.D., L.Ac., has integrated numerous wholistic medical techniques for the treatment of his patients. Dr. Ray says, "I began using olive leaf extract half a year ago, for parasites in particular. I have my patients open two capsules. They drop the powdered extract into a glass of water, and put in five to seven drops of deuterium sulphate.

"When one mixes any substance with deuterium sulphate and ingests the combination, there is evidence by microscopy that the resulting mixture penetrates human body cells within twelve hours. The deuterium sulphate, which is derived from that form of hydrogen known as *heavy water,* acts as a chemical substance delivery system to the cells," adds Dr. Ray.

"The somewhat acidifying olive leaf extract is excellent as treatment for my patients suffering with parasites, whose toxins cause them to be alkaline. Using the olive leaf powder, I've had increased success for people following my antiparasitic program," he advises. "When the olive leaf product first came out, the suggested dosage was one capsule twice daily, but I found that small a dose didn't do anything much. With the patients taking two or three pills three times a day, I'm experiencing a much better result for them. There will then be quick symptomatic relief of parasitic disease.

"Also added to the olive leaf extract are certain gentle herbs that come from my herbal manufacturing company. Together, they kill all known parasites. I'm not convinced that the olive leaf components alone kill the parasites themselves but rather they focus their killing power on the parasitic eggs and on the virus that travels inside each parasite's body," Dr. Ray states.

"Olive leaf extract is definitely one of the best natural products working effectively as a parasiticide. I have a positive impression of its ingredients' effectiveness. My patients with parasites are all getting better from taking olive leaf extract," says Dr. Timothy Ray.

The Nastiness of Human Parasites

Intestinal parasites have existed since our evolution as Homo sapiens, yet they were recognized as medical entities only within the last two hundred years. These protozoa and helminth worms may even have been a factor in Darwinian selection. They cause severe gastrointestinal symptoms, chief among them being diarrhea. The midafternoon siesta practiced in Latin American societies is possibly a cultural manifestation of unnatural lethargy caused by gastrointestinal invasion of these parasitic organisms.[1]

Diarrheal diseases are a primary cause of infant mortality. Those babies with strong immune systems and better nutrition survive, but many of the infected children reaching adulthood may never recognize a normal bowel movement or realize their full energy potential.

Parasites, by virtue of their nastiness, have attracted much attention among physicians and health care scientists, and now consumers have become aware of the invasive problem they face. Suddenly most of us know that one should not only be concerned with the dilemma of "guess what came to dinner," but also who prepared that dinner, where they prepared it, and how they went about the preparation of not only dinner, but also breakfast, lunch, and snacks as well. Chefs, short-order cooks, waiters, busboys, other restaurant workers, and householders who prepare meals are frequently the source of spreading parasitic infections. The presence of pets in the home is a polluting factor too.[2]

The Vastness of Your Gastrointestinal Tract

Spread flat, the surface area of one's gastrointestinal tract is the size of a football field and represents the most intimate interface between a human being and his or her environment. It's not surprising, therefore, that events which occur on the interior lining of the mouth, throat, stomach, and intestines (collectively known as the *gastrointestinal mucosa*) have effects upon the whole person.

These gastrointestinal mucosa and the long, narrow, tube-like channel they surround (the lumen) together form an enormously complex and dynamic ecosystem. The ecosystem furnishes a home for indigenous flora (microbial associates consisting of viruses, plants, and animals) which jointly constitute a major component. There are additional components including foods, other ingesta (solid or liquid nutrients) entering the lumen through the mouth, and one's body secretions that flow in by a variety of routes located along the mucosa. At any moment in time, this ecosystem reflects the equilibria existing among the channel's multiple components—most of them being beneficial but some causing harm to the human host. The various extra components might comprise billions of microbes both friendly and unfriendly, minerals, foreign substances, digestive enzymes, immune system constituents such as white blood cells, mucous production, ingesta, toxins, synthetics, pollutants, metallic particles, and a great deal more. Variations in these factors and the nutritional status of each person tends to affect an individual's intestinal environment and consequently the flora composition.

Interspersed among the lumen's flora are certain microscopic plants and animals—scavengers and predators—that obtain food at the expense of others. Sometimes these scavenger and/or predator organisms function within the human host symbiotically and at other times commensally. In a relationship known as *symbiosis,* there is an intimate and obligatory association between the two different species, the human and the microorganism. They are *symbionts* in which there is mutual aid and benefit between them. As stated in previous chapters, in a relationship referred to as *commensalism,* the microorganism lives in close association with the host and neither harms nor benefits it. For example, some flora living in the human gut obtain both food and a suitable habitat for themselves without hurting or giving any advantage to the individual.

Then there are parasites which live in a type of negative symbiotic relationship. In this case, the host is to some degree injured through the activities of the parasitic microorganism during the course of their intimate and protracted association. Some of the lumen's organisms have a changing interaction with their host's mucosa; sometimes the relationship is parasitic and sometimes it is commensal.

The Prevalence of Parasites

As defined in Chapter 10, a *parasite* is any living thing that flourishes within (an *endoparasite*) or upon (an *ectoparasite*) another living organism (the host). The parasite, which may spend all or only part of its existence with the host, obtains food and/or shelter from the host and contributes nothing to its welfare. Some parasites harm their hosts by causing irritation and interfering with bodily functions; others destroy host tissues and release toxins into the body, thus injuring health and causing disease. Human parasites which make themselves part of the gastrointestinal flora include viruses, fungi, bacteria, protozoa, and helminth worms.

Protozoa, which are nothing more than microparasites like viruses and bacteria, represent single cell *animal* organisms measuring from 1 to 10 millimeters (mm) in length. They multiply within their human hosts. The *helminth worms,* which are macroparasites of much larger size, grow as multicellular organisms but do *not* multiply inside their human hosts. Few people realize the enormous adverse impact these two types of parasites have on human well-being. They are the sources of serious diarrheal diseases worldwide and constitute the greatest single cause of sickness (morbidity) and death (mortality) for humankind. Numerous scientific studies have shown parasitic infection incidences ranging up to 99 percent of the populations in undeveloped countries. In the United States diarrheal diseases caused by intestinal infections are the third leading cause of morbidity and mortality.

Martin J. Lee, Ph.D., and Stephen Barrie, N.D., the two principal microbiologists of the Great Smokies Diagnostic Laboratory of Asheville, North Carolina, offer much information about the present generation of Americans, who have grown up with many modern sanitary conveniences. In the United States we assume that parasitic infections are encountered only in distant parts of the world or by people in impoverished rural areas. But Drs. Lee and Barrie cite authorities who say that Americans can acquire worm and protozoa invaders without doing any traveling, or even filing a passport application.

Signs, Symptoms, and Illnesses of Parasitic Infections

Parasite screening procedures using a series of laboratory tests taken by a physician with knowledge of parasitology will probably uncover the majority of parasitic organisms affecting humans. However, the signs and symptoms by themselves often are indicative of a parasite illness. The following are warning signs for the presence of parasites, either protozoa or helminths: constipation, diarrhea, gas and bloating, irritable bowel syndrome, joint and muscle aches and pains, anemia, allergy, skin conditions, granulomas, nervousness, sleep disturbances, teeth grinding, chronic fatigue, and immune system dysfunction.

Table 11 offers a listing of signs, symptoms, and illnesses of parasitic infections, especially those affecting the gastrointestinal tract, that will help you determine if there has been infestation by protozoa and/or helminthic worms.

A Microbiologist's Recovery from Malaria

On January 14, 1997, I received a telephone call from Mirium Rosallo, Ph.D., of Humble, Texas. Dr. Rosallo is a microbiologist working in the hemotology laboratory of the University of Texas Health Science Center at Houston. She had just learned from a university colleague, whom I had quoted in an earlier chapter, that I was gathering information for writing a book about olive leaf extract. Dr. Rosallo wanted to tell me her story of recovery from malaria as a result of using olive leaf extract after all other treatments had failed.

The woman first contracted this disease in 1979, at age eighteen, when she had been given a high school graduation gift of a safari in Kenya and Tanzania. ''I remember the setting in Mwanabwito, Tanzania, when I was bitten one

TABLE 11

Symptoms, Signs, and Illnesses of Parasitic Infections

Check yourself against this listing and see if you are affected by any of these difficulties related to protozoa and/or helminthic worms.

Anorexia	Arthritis
Autoimmune disease	Bloody stools
Chronic abdominal pain and cramps	Chronic fatigue
Colitis	Constipation
Crohn's disease	
Depressed secretory immunoglobulin A readings	Diarrhea
Distention of the abdomen	Dysentery
Fever	Flatulence
Food allergy	Foul-smelling stools
Gastritis	Headaches
Inflammatory bowel disease	
Increased or decreased intestinal permeability	Irregular bowel movements
Irritable bowel disease	
Leukopenia	Low back pain
Malabsorption	Pruritus ani
Rash and itching of the skin	Rectal bleeding
Urticaria	Vomiting
Weight loss	

night by *Anopheles bifurcatus,* the malaria mosquito,'' Mirium Rosallo said to me. ''As pre-exposure protection before and during the trip I took mefloquine [an antimalaria drug] once a week while in Africa, but it proved not to have been preventive for me. So as a preteen I came down with the symptoms of malaria: a periodic flu-like illness, aching muscles, nausea, coughing, fever that lasted for five hours and then dropped, chills, sweats, and headaches in cycles.

"Blood tests and blood counts were taken when I returned to the United States, and the malaria parasite, *Plasmodium falciparum,* was detected in blood smears placed on slides. I was diagnosed with the disease and hospitalized. My treatment included more antimalarial drugs in varying combinations and doses, intravenous fluids, and even red blood cell transfusions," Dr. Rosallo explained. "Still, periodically—maybe every few months—I went through relapses and experienced the symptoms once again."

Malaria is a serious infection caused by one or more of at least four different species of the protozoan organism *Plasmodium,* transferred by a mosquito vector. It leads to chills, fever, anemia, and an enlarged spleen (among other symptoms). Malaria tends to become a lifelong disease, and it's carried from human to human by a bite from an infected female *Anopheles* mosquito which sucks animal or human blood to feed her eggs. The disease is also spread by blood transfusion or by the use of an infected needle, and is often found among intravenous drug users who share needles.

Plasmodium parasites enter the red blood cells of the infected human, where they mature, reproduce, and burst out every so often. Malaria attacks (paroxysms) occur at regular intervals. They go together with the growth of new parasites in the body. Bouts of malaria usually last from one to four weeks, but attacks occur less often as the disease continues. Still, insecticide-immune mosquitoes and drug-resistant protozoa have developed, and malaria continues to be a danger worldwide. Between 300 million and 500 million people now get malaria each year, and someone dies of it about every fifteen seconds—mostly children and pregnant women. Over the last decade, malaria has killed about ten times as many children as all wars around our planet in that same period.[3]

"On September 26, 1996, my symptoms of acute fatigue and weakness, to the point of complete collapse, caused my

husband to take me to the nearest hospital emergency room,"
continued Dr. Rosallo. "The physician on duty there found
that I had too little oxygen in my blood and a white blood
cell [WBC] count of over 24,000. (Normal for a healthy
female is about 7,000 WBCs per cubic millimeter of blood.) I
was hospitalized and given antibiotics, steroids (prednisone),
plus other drugs. My regular physician was looking for some
type of viral invasion, and didn't consider these symptoms
part of my original malarial infestation. The drugs she had
administered only seemed to make my condition worse. She
kept saying to my relatives, 'I don't know what to do; Mirium
has a viral infection and we can't find it.' Then she would
go on to try some other drug on me.

"My white blood cells would drop off slowly and then
shoot back up to 24,000. I was getting no better, so my
mother contacted a friend of ours, Eve Coombs, who coun-
sels in the nutrition field, in an area just north of Toronto.
In conjecturing that my symptoms could be connected with
malaria, Eve suggested I try olive leaf extract. My mother
brought it into the hospital, and I took two capsules every
day for four days. Even with just the first two capsules, my
body responded amazingly fast. The hospital nurses were
keeping track of my urine and blood test readings, and the
olive leaf extract caused me to eliminate all kinds of parasites, of course including the *Plasmodium,* which they could
see under the microscope. Since I'm a working microbiologist, the technicians gave me the courtesy of looking through
the scope to view my own organisms.

"My WBC count dropped a little every day to reach the
normal range, until I was released from the hospital completely
free of illness on October 7, 1996. My WBC count continues
to remain regulated to this day," acknowledged Dr. Rosallo.
"I take two capsules of olive leaf extract each day to prevent
a return bout of malaria. My sense is that if I don't use the
olive leaf product on a regular basis, malarial symptoms will
come back. It truly fights off parasites."

❧

CHAPTER 13

Concluding Information for Successfully Using Olive Leaf Extract

Wilford Bruno Graciano, the fifty-four-year-old executive vice president and chief operating officer (COO) of ConMac Securities, Inc., a Wall Street investment management firm, began to have health problems. He was experiencing periodic episodes of palsy-like tremors in both of his hands, accompanied by weakness of the arms so severe he could hardly lift them to button his shirt collar or hold a phone to his ear. During March 1996, the COO was also troubled by an unrelenting tic-like blinking of the left eye, a shuffling gait, constant low-grade fever, and a chronic gnawing headache. His family physician could reach no conclusion about these problems, so she sent her patient for consultation with a prominent university-affiliated neurologist.

After undergoing a detailed history-taking, a thorough clinical examination, and numerous laboratory tests, Mr. Graciano was referred by the neurologist for magnetic resonance imaging (MRI). The MRI was not a usual one, for it involved the injection of gadolinium, a paramagnetic contrast agent for color viewing the interior of his brain and spinal cord. When the results arrived, the neurologist saw his patient again. "You probably have been affected by a perivascular central nervous system demyelination,'' the specialist said, but the executive didn't understand this diagnosis. Therefore, it was further described as a kind of ''neuroparalytic accident,'' not a brain tumor and not connected with any bacterial disease but possibly originating from a viral infection. The diagnosis remained uncertain because the virus had not been identified.

''There isn't much to be done to correct the problem,'' said the neurologist, ''but I'll confer with your physician to see if we can come up with some kind of treatment plan. Goodbye and good luck! On your way out, please see my receptionist to make payment.'' The nerve specialist's examination fee plus the laboratory tests and MRI came to $3,250, of which Wilford Graciano's health insurance carrier paid a fractional amount.

The patient's family physician admitted that she didn't know how to proceed. A subsequent telephone conference she undertook with the neurologist failed to offer any clearcut treatment procedure. ''Maybe you ought to consult somebody else,'' the doctor said later.

Difficulties with Accessing Medical Information Online

Now Mr. Graciano had not reached his executive position in finance by being forsaken or otherwise sloughed off by anyone, even by his family doctor or a professor of neurology. His highly lucrative business career, prolonged good health, and life expectancy were being jeopardized, the executive realized. So he decided to do a lot more investigating to learn exactly what ailed him and the steps for bringing about bodily repair. That's when he decided to access medical information online. He was determined to become an educated patient and empower himself in clinical terms by finding health options through research by computer.

He also consulted another neurological specialist. He set

up an appointment for a fuller set of diagnostic procedures with another New York City neurologist, who agreed to hospitalize him at the Mount Sinai Medical Center for four days of testing. The hospitalization was to occur a month hence.

Meantime, he assigned a securities analyst member of his office staff to research online accurate, timely, and appropriate information about his symptoms and their source. The employee used all the information technologies available to the company. Though ConMac Securities, Inc. regularly deals with national businesses, worldwide industries, investment securities, international banking, and other complex forms of commerce, she discovered that her procedures did not work!

The staff member explained to her boss that the difficulties of accessing medical information online were overwhelming. It takes special training to cope with health information technologies. The medical and computer terminology combined present problems. It was beyond her computer skills to accomplish these tasks.

Quite simply, patients and other medical consumers have too little information for acquiring successful health care. In contrast, physicians and other health care practitioners generally get too much informational input. Medical material must be expanded for consumers and summarized for medical personnel.

Particularly vexing are the many frustrations encountered by needy participants like Wilford Graciano. They are due to current information systems' failure to furnish knowledge that can be easily accessible. Poor information flow has become an impediment to efficient delivery of high-quality diagnoses and treatment.

Most of the clinical, administrative, and educational material that flows throughout the health care system continues to be recorded on paper. Over 10 billion pages of patient records are produced in the United States each year, each of them a masterpiece of idiosyncratic functionality. If online services did not exist, much written material would be lost to the medical community at large, and progress in health care would proceed at the snail's pace it has up to now—at least until computers are employed by medically knowledgeable personnel.[1]

Wilford Graciano Receives a Diagnosis and "Treatment" of Sorts

For twenty workdays Wilford Graciano's employee searched by computer for sources of information in various fields of medicine. She tapped into the vast online storehouse of medical and health information via the Internet, commercial online services, and bulletin board systems. Unfortunately for her employer, although the computer operator did produce a high pile of health information printouts, she did not know how to classify them. Her search had netted much miscellaneous information but none of it was helpful to Mr. Graciano, because it was nonspecific. A difficulty here was that the patient had no true diagnosis on which one could focus. The employee didn't know the appropriate key words to base her search on.

The time came for Mr. Graciano to take four days off and enter the Mount Sinai Hospital's diagnostic testing program. Mr. Graciano did it with reluctance, because he knew that much business income would be lost in his absence. But his physical abilities were becoming limited. He could no longer pick up a pen, even to sign his name, he didn't wear a tie because he was unable to fashion a knot, and he stopped going to lunch with clients since his left eye tic had him winking at them all the time. The only thing Mr. Graciano did well was show anger and irritability by shouting, screaming, and making demands. He apologized for his behavior but continued to act as the office tyrant. His employees were overjoyed when their boss left for four days to seek diagnosis, treatment, and perhaps a cure.

As it turned out, the doctors kept Mr. Graciano hospitalized for a full week, at the end of which he was given a diagnosis of sorts, but his condition was nontreatable. The patient was told that he did not suffer from Parkinson's disease (PD), multiple sclerosis (MS), amyotrophic lateral sclerosis (ALS), central nervous system neoplasm, or any other such neurological disease of the brain and spinal cord. Rather, his spinal cord cells were invaded by one of the thirty-six serotypes of a relatively rare echovirus causing chronic aseptic meningitis. This is a viral infection which could send him into a coma or actually threaten his life. If so, coma or death could strike within a few months or weeks.

Antibiotics are not only worthless against viral infections in general, but particularly are poor treatment for chronic aseptic meningitis, because the rare echovirus affecting him thrived on such drugs. The doctors named it "a superbug," the type of individual viral organism (the virion) which utilizes antibiotics as nourishment. Subsequently they offered another suggestion for treatment.

Side Effects of Treatment with Acyclovir

Although it has never been found useful against echoviruses, the only therapy possible, assured the hospital's physician and his attending neurologist, was high dosage acyclovir. Acyclovir, a white sterile powder brandnamed Zovirax®, has been utilized to relieve the symptoms of, but not cure, genital herpes virus infections and mucocutaneous herpes simplex virus infections. The herpes virus is a different species from the echovirus form producing chronic aseptic meningitis.

For treatment of Mr. Graciano's disease, it would be risky to employ acyclovir, admitted the doctors, inasmuch as an elevated intravenous (IV) quantity of the medication was required. IV acyclovir had to be given slowly, over not less than a one-hour period; otherwise, dire consequences would ensue. Additionally, Mr. Graciano needed a minimum acyclovir dosage of 10 milligrams per kilogram of body weight (10 mg/kg) administered IV every eight hours, which had to be started promptly, the physicians advised, and continued at least ten days for its maximal therapeutic benefit.

But then the patient learned that IV acyclovir has numerous adverse side effects. Not only can it cause pain on urination, abdominal pain, fever, phlebitis, inflammation, blood vessel obstruction, nausea, vomiting, itching, rash, hives, lethargy, psychosis, tremors, hallucinations, confusion, lightheadedness, agitation, and seizures, but it has also produced the more dangerous symptoms of abnormal liver function, bone marrow suppression, blood in the urine, anemia, and transient kidney failure. Moreover, the drug itself, when given IV, has been a source of coma and anaphylaxis resulting in death.

Wilford Graciano wanted none of these additional disorders. Being a decisive individual all of his life, he refused further testing and signed out of the medical center without any treatment. The ConMac executive didn't know what to do next, but he was determined that drug therapy would not be what eventually killed him.

Grandma Graciano Brings Willy Olive Leaf Extract

His bad news was devastating to family, friends, professional colleagues, and coworkers. Consequently, the very next Sunday, the entire Graciano clan living in America gathered from far and wide and paid their respects to their most successful member. His father's mother, Grandma Rose Graciano, then ninety-eight years old, demanded that she be taken to visit him. In the confines of her grandson's twenty-eight-room mansion, located in affluent Greenwich, Connecticut, she talked persuasively in Italian to Wilford Graciano.

In part Grandma Graciano said, "Willy, do you remember when you were a small boy and you lived in my house in Little Italy with your mommy and daddy? Do you remember that every day I would give you a light green drink to keep you healthy?"

Sitting in dazed disbelief at the death sentence facing him, knee to knee before his grandmother, Wilford Graciano shook his head affirmatively. "I do remember, Grandma. It had a bitter taste, but I drank down what you gave to me because I love you."

"Well, this drink was created from leaves of 'the tree of life.' And it prevented you from ever getting colds or flu or any other kind of infection. Do you remember that, Willy? You never became sick, except if you went on some trip without drinking it. Then you came home with a cold, but the green drink would cure that cold overnight. Do you agree?"

"Yes, Grandma," Wilford Graciano said, "but a drink made from leaves of the olive tree won't cure the bad germs that I've got now."

"But it will, Willy, and I've brought you a few jars right here in this bag. Please, Willy, you were the tiny baby I helped to bring into this world, and I ask you to please let me try to keep you in this world a little longer. Please, because you love me, drink this olive leaf liquid every day. Each week I will send over more jars for you. Please drink a jar a day. Will you do that for me, Willy?" asked Grandma Graciano.

Out of consideration for his much loved grandmother, Wilford Graciano promised that he would drink an eight-ounce jar of olive leaf extract every day, divided into four ounces in the morning and four ounces in the evening. And he's alive today, feeling healthy, happy, and grateful to his grandmother for being persistent. He continues to take olive leaf extract daily, only in a more convenient capsular form.

For at least the last four thousand years, populations in countries bordering the Mediterranean, where olive trees grow abundantly, have swallowed chopped up olive leaves in liquid or salad form as a supplement to their diets to prevent or treat microbial infections.

It was only by a lucky accident that Wilford Bruno Graciano had his life saved (and perhaps even improved) through the loving persistence of his ninety-eight-year-old grandmother who recognized the antimicrobial attributes of drinking an extract made from olive leaves.

The Action of Olive Leaf Extract on Microbes

A leaflet distributed by James R. Privitera, M.D., of Covina, California, explains the product's natural herbal action. Dr. Privitera explains, "Olive leaf extract has a number of unique properties that help destroy viruses, bacteria, and parasites. It interferes with critical amino acid production essential for viruses, and has the ability to contain viral infection and/or spread by inactivating viruses or by preventing virus shedding, budding or assembling at the cell membranes. It directly penetrates infected cells and stops viral replication. In the case of retroviruses, olive leaf extract is able to neutralize the production of reverse transcriptase and protease. These enzymes are essential for a retrovirus, such as HIV, to alter the RNA of a healthy cell. It can stimulate phagocytosis, an immune system response in which cells ingest harmful microorganisms and foreign matter."

Dr. Privitera went on to say, "Olive leaf extract may possess powerful antioxidant properties. It has been shown to inhibit oxidation of low-density lipoproteins, the so-called 'bad cholesterol' involved in heart and arterial disease. Moreover, it's effective in combating a wide range of health problems as well as serving as a preventative against illness. With its antioxidant properties, olive leaf extract has great potential as an adjunct for people involved in vigorous exercise programs in order to stop the generation of free radicals and the resulting damage they cause to healthy cells.''

Going on to list some of the most obvious advantages to people taking the herbal product, Dr. Privitera says, ''Olive leaf extract has been reported to:

- enhance the immune system,[2]
- increase energy,
- offer an internal cleansing action,
- be antiviral, antifungal, antibacterial, and antiparasitic,[3]
- lower elevated blood pressure for hypertensives,[4]
- protect against the oxidation of low density lipoprotein,[5]
- reduce, ameliorate or even eliminate many diverse health problems [fibromyalgia, psoriasis, cardiomyopathy, and more].

''Olive leaf extract is the rediscovery of a substance used in Biblical times,'' continues Dr. Privitera. ''The ancient Egyptians may have been the first to make practical application of it, for the mummification of their pharaohs. In later cultures, olive leaf extracts were used as a popular folk remedy to relieve fevers. A simple healing remedy using olive leaves was published in 1854 in the *Pharmaceutical Journal*. More recently, Italian researchers found oleuropein had the capacity to lower blood pressure in animals. Other European researchers confirmed this finding and determined that it also increased blood flow in the coronary arteries, relieved arrhythmias, and prevented intestinal muscle spasms.

''In the late 1960s, research by The Upjohn Pharmaceutical Company showed that elenolic acid, a substance derived from olive leaf extract, killed every virus tested—every one! Among those viruses tested were herpes, influenza, a couple of leukemias, and a sarcoma. It was found to counteract a variety of viruses associated with the common cold in humans. Furthermore, elenolic acid was also effective against parasitic protozoans and bacteria,'' concluded Dr. Privitera.

Olive Leaves Send Enzymes Against Recognized Microbes

Olive leaves and other plants recognize disease-causing microbes and produce an antimicrobial enzyme called *Pto kinase,* a protein. This finding was uncovered by Gregory B. Martin, associate professor of agronomy at Purdue University. Pto kinase is produced by a disease-resistance gene in olive leaves and certain other plants. It kills off microbes, particularly bacteria, by binding to a protein produced by disease-causing microorganisms, which alert the plants' various defense mechanisms.

''It turns out that plants resist diverse pathogens—including bacteria, fungi, and viruses—by using very similar defense mechanisms,'' Dr. Martin says. ''By understanding how a plant recognizes one pathogen, we should begin to understand how plants identify many different pathogens.''

The discovery of this protein-protein interaction was reported in the December 20, 1996, issue of *Science,* and the same issue contained a second research paper that addressed different aspects of the recognition mechanism, which was written by researchers from the laboratory of Brian Staskawicz, professor of plant biology at the University of California, Berkeley.

''The field of plant disease resistance has just crystallized in the past two to three years,'' Dr. Martin says. ''It has become one of the fastest-moving areas of plant biology.''[6]

Since the 1940s, when a scientist named H. H. Flor first proposed that disease resistance in plants like olive trees requires both a dominant resistance gene in the plant and a dominant gene in the pathogen, scientists have struggled to determine if Dr. Flor's "gene-for-gene" theory was correct and how it might work.

In 1993, Dr. Martin was successful in cloning the first disease-resistance gene in crop plants, named *Pto,* which is involved in gene-for-gene disease resistance. But the agronomist and his colleagues at Purdue struggled to understand the molecular mechanism of disease resistance. One puzzle was why the protein that provides resistance to infection is found *inside* the cells instead of *on* the cell walls, where one would expect a defense mechanism to be. Then the "type III secretion pathway" was revealed to them. This type III secretion pathway is used by microbes when they infect cells, not by invading the cell wall, but by introducing proteins directly into the host cell's cytoplasm. The protein introduction alerts the plants' various defense systems and causes their release of "avirulence" genes, or *avrPto,* which alert the resistance plants' defense mechanisms.

Olive leaf extract is theorized to work, in part, because it contains stored avrPto. Thus avrPto is always at the ready to provide a microcidal effect against pathological organisms.

Efficacy of Olive Leaf Tincture Against Herpes

Writing in the "Letters to the Editor" column of the May 1997 *Townsend Letter for Doctors & Patients,* William R. Fredrickson of Indianapolis, Indiana, who conducted research on olive leaf extract, reports on the efficacy of *Tinctura Olea Foliorum,* an olive leaf preparation provided as a tincture (an alcoholic concentrate made from the tree's olive leaves). The tincture, which dates back to 1827, when the hydro-ethanolic extract of olive leaves was used for the treatment of malaria, is made by boiling olive leaves in water, creating an aqueous extract which is combined with wine. Then and later, as well, in 1854 and 1906, this preparation was acknowledged to be superior to quinine in the treatment of malarial infection.

Mr. Fredrickson takes credit for discovering that subtle structural changes in the active molecule of olive leaves (oleuropein) significantly lessens the binding of serum proteins. Serum protein binding was the biochemical problem unsolved by The Upjohn Company, which caused them to drop olive leaf extract as a viable antimicrobial product. Such structural changes take place naturally when someone employs *Tinctura Olea Foliorum* as the effective therapeutic agent against infections of various types.

Research on *Tinctura Olea Foliorum* was conducted by Leslie Nachman, the present vice president of East Park Research, Inc. of Henderson, Nevada, and Robert B. Strecker, M.D., Ph.D., of Eagle Rock, California. Dr. Strecker is a practicing gastroenterologist and internist with training in pathology and his Ph.D. is in pharmacology.

Nachman and Strecker marketed *Tinctura Olea Foliorum* under the name *Viliv*.™ During March 1993, they set up a study with a physician, Jerry Ponitch, M.D., of Tempe, Arizona, to test the efficacy of Viliv™ against herpectic infection. Six men and women from Dr. Ponitch's practice were chosen who had periodically shown infections with herpes simplex virus type II (genital herpes) and probably herpes simplex virus type I. The lesions of herpes simplex 1 appear as small fluid-filled vesicles with raised red bases on the skin and mucous membranes in nongenital areas.

Dr. Ponitch drew blood from the six people and sent it to the Metwest Clinical Laboratory in Phoenix, Arizona, to determine each person's initial antibody level to the herpes virus. The patients were then required to take two ounces of Viliv™ every six hours. After some days elapsed, all the patients reported experiencing relief from their herpes lesions, and three reported the disappearance of them in thirty-six to forty-eight hours.

One of the other three subjects, a thirty-four-year-old woman, had several months earlier discontinued her use of the birth control pill. She subsequently experienced estrogen surges which suppressed her immunity, and may have been responsible for her contracting genital herpes. The physician put the woman on four ounces of *Tinctura Olea Foliorum* to be taken every six hours. She reported that almost all of her lesions were gone three days later.

The two remaining patients, a man and woman, were newly infected with herpes genitalis and experiencing a much higher level of viral shedding. Taking four ounces of Viliv™ every six hours, the lesions causing them discomfort disappeared quickly.

All six subjects reported that the tincture of olive leaf extract worked considerably better for them than acyclovir, the medication they had been prescribed. No other medications were prescribed by Dr. Ponitch during his study, and any other medication his patients had been taking, such as aloe vera extract, the amino acid lysine, and additional nutritional supplements, had been discontinued by them at least one week before the study began. All subjects reported the presence of herpes lesions at the start of this study.

Description of the Herpes Study Procedure

"The primary objective [of the herpes study] was to lessen or eliminate the severity of the lesions and their accompanying pain. Successful completion of this task was taken as one of the end points of the study," Mr. William Frederickson told the *Townsend Letter* editor.

"Then a secondary object was to try and lower serum antibody levels the herpes virus. Significant reduction of greater than 50 percent was taken to be a sign of measured lowering of the viral load upon the immune system. The individual subject's blood was checked for levels of Herpes 1 and 2 antibodies (IgM; one subject had IgM and IgG) before the study began. Antibody levels were then checked at two weeks," writes Mr. Frederickson.[7]

The result was that three of the infected people reported being able to eat foods which normally made them break out in herpes lesions, arginine-rich foods such as pork, corn, onions, etc. When taking the tincture, the patients reported no outbreaks to such foods. *Tinctura Olea Foliorum* is at least as effective as acyclovir in controlling herpetic infection (if not more so). All of the people involved expressed happiness with the tincture, and according to their comments, it's superior to acyclovir in controlling genital herpes. Antibody levels in one of the subjects decreased by 22.8 percent, an indication that the herpes infection itself may be cast off from the victim's cells.

The Rising Tide of Treatment-Resistant Fungi

Like bacteria, pathogenic fungi have proven to be consummate opportunists, readily invading relatively new immunosuppressed populations in hospitals and the community. These are people with immune systems weakened by AIDS, aggressive cancer chemotherapy or drugs aimed at foiling rejection of transplanted organs. While immunocompromised people are most at risk, disease-causing fungi pose a threat to the rest of us as well, particularly when the microbes are resistant to antifungal agents. Otherwise healthy patients hospitalized for elective surgery, for example, are potential prey for fungi transmitted through catheters, prostheses, and other invasive devices.

Studies confirm a surge in the rates of nosocomial fungal infections. According to a review of data from 115 sentinel hospitals by the Centers for Disease Control and Prevention's National Nosocomial Infections Surveillance System, the proportion of hospital-acquired infections caused by fungi (mainly *Candida albicans*) nearly doubled from 1980 to 1990, from 6 percent to 11 percent.

Although scientists and physicians have fretted over the

seemingly diabolical ability of bacteria to evolve strategies for outmaneuvering antibiotics, pathogenic fungi using similar tactics are now also registering resistance to treatment. Fungal infections have been on the rise during the past twenty years. The emergence more recently of fungi that are resistant to the modest arsenal of drugs used to treat them has raised the specter of the fungal equivalent of multidrug-resistant bacteria.

"While we've become accustomed to appreciating the problems of antibacterial resistance, this level of resistance by fungi to antifungal drugs is historically unprecedented," says Thomas J. Walsh, M.D., head of the immunocompromised host division of the National Cancer Institute (NCI) of Bethesda, Maryland.

"Just five to ten years ago, textbooks said the emergence of resistance to antifungals is a rare event. Now it is a cause of great concern," Dr. Walsh told a symposium on antifungal drug resistance convened at the 36th Interscience Conference on Antimicrobial Agents and Chemotherapy, held in New Orleans.[8]

Natural Olive Leaf Extract Supersedes Synthetic Antifungal Drugs

The antifungal pharmacopeia, including the newest agents developed during the last decade, such as the triazoles (fluconazole, ketoconazole, and itraconazole), 5-fluorocytosine (5-FC), and amphotericin B, are inadequate to handle the rising tide of resistant fungi. There's too massive an increase in the incidence of such fungal infections. Physicians' heavy reliance on these mainstays to prevent or treat such disease entities in patients with AIDS, cancer victims undergoing chemotherapy, and others with impaired immunity has encouraged the fungal pathogens to evolve methods to elude the synthetic antifungal drugs.

"Unfortunately, the fungi have learned to respond to this

increasing antifungal pressure, and we have seen a change in our ability to treat infections such as oropharyngeal candidiasis [thrush], for which AIDS patients are at substantial risk," says John H. Rex, M.D., of the University of Texas Medical School at Houston who, with Dr. Walsh, convened the New Orleans Interscience symposium. "We've seen a change in our ability to treat fungal infections of all kinds."

Unlike bacteria, Fungi have chromosomes, cells with a true nucleus bounded by a nuclear membrane, and exhibit mitosis. Because their cellular structure is so similar to our own, it is difficult to develop drugs that inhibit their growth without unacceptable toxicity. Synthetic antifungal drugs coming out of the laboratories of pharmaceutical companies are just too poisonous to use. Their adverse side effects are overwhelming.

In contrast, olive leaf extract is nontoxic in the recommended dosages. This natural product discovers the chinks in the fungal microbes' armor and exploits them. One finding that has emerged from research on fungal resistance is that these microorganisms differ from bacteria by behaving more like cancer cells that develop resistance to antineoplastic agents.

"So far, we have found three mechanisms, all of which are strikingly analogous to those of cancer cells," explains Dr. Walsh. "The fungal cells literally pump the drug back out of themselves. In others, the fungi render the drug impotent by either mutating or producing overwhelming amounts of the [fungal] target of the drug."

Nearly all the synthetic drugs are fungistatic in their actions; that is, when they're working, they inhibit the growth of fungi. Olive leaf extract is different; most of the time its fungicidal. It has the ability to kill the invading fungus rather than merely inhibiting its growth. As a fungicidal drug, olive leaf extract offers the advantage of leaving behind fewer fungal cells, thus lowering the potential of a drug-resistant mutation. This antimicrobial attribute reduces the likelihood of relapse after stopping therapy with olive leaf extract.

Since not all patients respond to antifungal drugs, even when the infecting organism is not a drug-resistant strain, boosting host immunity becomes important as another antifungal strategy. Olive leaf extract does that too. It buys such patients time. Of course, if immunosuppressed patients are not ultimately able to organize a good defense, they may succumb to the fungus infection.

Researchers speculate that a subtle deficiency of the immune system may explain why some apparently healthy people who contract fungal infections such as coccidioidomycosis or histoplasmosis develop severe, fulminant, and sometimes fatal infections, while most people respond to olive leaf extract and recover.

A P P E N D I X

❧

Product Distributors and Information Resources

Olive Leaf Extract

- EAST PARK RESEARCH, Inc., manufacturer and distributor of American made olive leaf extract, President Gordon G. Melcher and Vice President Leslie Nachman, P.O. Box 530099, Henderson, Nevada 89053 or 1777 Crystal Stream Avenue, Henderson, Nevada 89012; telephone (702) 837-1111; teleFAX (702) 837-1110. To place an order for this patented, encapsulated olive leaf product brandnamed, East Park™ Olive Leaf Extract, telephone tollfree to (800) 345-8367.
- NEW ACTION PRODUCTS, President Rose Emerson, 147 Ontario Street, Buffalo, New York 14207; telephone (716) 873-3738; FAX (716) 873-6621. To place an order for the encapsulated olive leaf product derived from East Park™ Olive Leaf Extract, telephone to the New Action Products' regular business number.
- GK PRODUCTS, Inc., President Ajit Channe, 10088 Northwest Third Place, Coral Springs, Florida 33071; telephone tollfree to (888) 752-4286; teleFAX (954)-752-4061; E-mail: ajeet@worldnet.att.net. To place an order for the encapsulated olive leaf product derived

from East Park™ Olive Leaf Extract, telephone to the GK Products, Inc. 888 number.

- AMERIHEALTH, President Richard L. Hall, P.O. Box 1870, Fallbrook, California 92088 or 4241 Via Eldorado, Fallbrook, California 92028; telephone (888) 405-3336; teleFAX (760) 728-0608; E-mail: richard@ amerihealth.com; website: www.2amerihealth.com is the provider of the encapsulated East Park™ Olive Leaf Extract brand and other nutritional supplements. To place an order, telephone to the tollfree number shown here.

- GREAT CONTINENTS INTERNATIONAL HOLDING COMPANY, parent of GCI NUTRIENTS, Inc., are raw materials suppliers, and manufacturers of the olive leaf extract brand known as *Olivir*™. This product is offered in bulk powder of 5% oleuropein, 500 mg tablets, and 500 mg capsules by the company's chief executive officer, Richard Merriam, or vice president, Michael J. Solomon, 1501 Adrian Road, Burlingame, California 94010; telephone (650) 697-4700; FAX (650) 697-6300. GCI NUTRIENTS, Inc., offers the Olivir™ brand of olive leaf extract to distributors, which is a trademark of BioStar Nutriceuticals, Inc., an affiliate.

- NUTRICOLOGY, Inc., d/b/a ALLERGY RESEARCH GROUP, Research Director Stephan A. Levine, Ph.D., 400 Preda Street, P.O. Box 489, San Leandro, California 94577-0489; tel. (510) 639-4572; FAX (510) 635-6730; to place an order for the private label olive leaf product, Prolive™ with Antioxidants, derived from the Olivir™ brand, telephone (800) 545-9960.

- IMMUNOSCREEN, President James R. Privitera, M.D., 105 North Grandview, Covina, California 91723; tel. (626) 966-1618; FAX (626) 966-7226; to place an order for the encapsulated, clinically proven olive leaf extracted product Olivex™, telephone (888) 220-7888.

- PROGRESSIVE LABORATORIES, Inc., President

Joe O'Neal and Marketing Director William Eicher, 1701 West Walnut Hill Lane, Irving, Texas 75038-7962; tel. (214) 518-9660; FAX (214) 518-9665; to order the olive leaf product, #837, Olivir™ Herbal Capsules, telephone (800) 527-9512.

- DOUGLAS LABORATORIES, President Douglas Lioon, 600 Boyce Road, Pittsburgh, Pennsylvania 15205; telephone (412) 494-0122 and in Europe (31)(0)455-444-777; FAX (412) 494-0155; to order the Olivir™ brand of olive leaf extract, telephone in the USA and Canada (800) 245-4440.

- NATURE'S PLUS, Inc., 548 Broadhollow Road, Melville, New York 11747. Nature's Plus manufactures Herbal Actives Olive Leaf Extract, a highly effective product, standardized at the preferred level of 6% oleuropein (see page 89–90). Cold processed, to ensure high activity, Herbal Actives Olive Leaf Extract also includes whole herb and the complete range of synergistic cofactors present in fresh herb. To find out where you can purchase Herbal Actives Olive Leaf Extract, please call 1(800) 645-9500.

- OPTIMAL NUTRIENTS, Inc., 1163 Chess Drive, Foster City, California 94404; FAX (415) 349-1686, to order the Olivir™ brand of olive leaf extract, telephone (800) 966-8874.

- PROGRESSIVE NUTRITION, Inc., 1860 Eastern Avenue, #106, Ventura, California 93003; to order the Olivir™ brand of olive leaf extract, telephone (805) 644-3023, FAX (805) 644-6079.

- LIFEWISE NATURALS, Inc., 375 Midway Circle, Nixa, Missouri 65714; telephone (417) 881-2561; tele-FAX (414) 725-9688. To order the Lifewise Naturals® Olivir™ brand of olive leaf extract, telephone tollfree (800) 643-9558.

- FOOD SCIENCE CORPORATION, 20 New England Drive, Essex Junction, Vermont 05452, telephone (802) 878-5508; FAX (802) 878-0549; distributes its brand of olive leaf extract, Olivir™, standardized to 15–25 percent oleuropein, through two divisions. Specifically for health professionals, order from Da Vinci Laboratories at (800) 325-1776. For the consumer, order from FoodScience Laboratories at (800) 874-9444.

- LIFE SECRETS, Inc., 37 Midland Avenue, Elmwood Park, New Jersey 07407; telephone (877) SECRET-9 (732-7389); FAX (877) 797-6180; to order O-live™ brand of olive leaf extract in tablet or capsule form or O-live™ Plus Gel for topical application, or O-live™ Plus Tablets or Capsules containing glucosamine, or O-live™ Deluxe containing glucosamine and chondroitin sulfate A & B, phone tollfree (800) 255-6679.

- EXTRACTSPLUS, Inc., 5800 Newton Drive, Carlsbad, California 92008; telephone (760) 431-8324; FAX (760) 431-8610; imports and wholesales bulk olive leaf powdered extract manufactured to pharmaceutical specifications by Flachsmann AG of Zurich, Switzerland. The bulk powder contains 17 to 23 percent oleuropein determined by the high-performance liquid chromatography (HPLC) testing method.

- ROEX, Inc., 2081 Business Center Drive, Suite #185, Irvine, California 92612 or mailing address: P.O. Box 19339, Irvine, California 92623; telephone (800) 645-0010 or (714) 476-8675; FAX (888) 329-7639 or (714) 476-8682; Homepage: http://roex.com; distributes Roex Oleuropein (Olive Leaf Extract) derived from the high potency ExtractsPlus, Inc. bulk import. Roex Oleuropein is available in bottles of 60 tablets of 250 milligrams of oleuropein. The recommended dosage of this 17–23% potent product is one tablet, one to four times per day preferably between meals.

- SOLARAY® HERBS, a division of NUTRACEUTICAL CORPORATION, 1500 Kearns Boulevard, Suite 200, Park City, Utah 84060 or mailing address P.O. Box 681869, Park City, Utah 84068; telephone (801) 655-6128; teleFax (801) 655-6029, sells olive leaf extract exclusively through independent health food stores. SOLARAY® Olive Leaf Extract capsules contain 250 mg. of the high-potency ExtractsPlus, Inc. olive leaf extract (17% to 23% oleuropein) plus 85 mg. of lemon balm leaf. Recommended dosage is one to four capsules daily. For a listing of stores retailing capsules containing Solaray® Olive Leaf Extract, contact the Nutraceutical Corporation toll-free at (800) 579-4665.

- M.W. INTERNATIONAL, Inc. is a raw material supplier of standardized Olive Leaf Extract produced with a minimum of 6 percent Oleuropein under GMP (Good Manufacturing Practices) guidelines. The company is located at 225 Long Avenue, P.O. Box 308, Hillside, New Jersey 07205. To place an order or for more information, telephone the Customer Service Department tollfree at (800) 371-7921 or (973) 926-4025 or teleFAX (973) 926-0989. Visit the M.W. International website at www.mwinternational.com

- SOURCE NATURALS, P.O. Box 2118, Santa Cruz, California 95063; telephone (800) 777-5677; teleFAX (408) 438-7410, Jeff Lipsuis, Vice President.

Sources of Loose Olive Leaves for Brewing Tea

If you have an olive tree of the manzanillo or mission green olive species growing in your neighborhood, you can pick the leaves right off the tree and use them for therapeutic purposes. Otherwise, wholesale purchases of olive leaves may be made from:

- SAN FRANCISCO HERB COMPANY, 47444 Kato Road, Fremont, California 94538; telephone (510) 770-1215, telefax (510) 770-9021. Ask for whole olive leaves *(Olea europaea)*—product number W1119. Alternatively, your local health food store may order olive leaves for you from the San Francisco Herb Company.

Infectious Disease Information

- CENTERS FOR DISEASE CONTROL AND PREVENTION (CDC); general telephone for any inquiry (404) 639-3311, voice mail (404) 639-3311, International Travel Directory (404) 332-4565, International Travelers' Hotline (404) 332-4559 and in Spanish (404) 330-3132.
- FOOD AND DRUG ADMINISTRATION; general telephone for any inquiry (301) 443-3170.
- NATIONAL INSTITUTES OF HEALTH, Informaton Office, Building 31, Room 7A32, Bethesda, Maryland 20892; telephone (800) 874-2572.
- AMERICAN SOCIAL HEALTH ASSOCIATION for Sexually Transmitted Diseases, P.O. Box 13827, Research Triangle Park, North Carolina 27709; telephone (800) 227-8922.

AIDS Organizations and Newsletters

- KEEP HOPE ALIVE, Executive Director & Newsletter Editor Mark Konlee, *Positive Health News*, P.O. Box 27041, West Allis, Wisconsin 53227; voice mail telephone (414) 548-4344; fax (414) 679-2885; web site: http://www.execpc.com/keephope/keephope.html.
- CDC NATIONAL AIDS CLEARINGHOUSE, P.O. Box 6003, Rockville, Maryland 20849-6003; telephone (800) 458-5231.
- CRITICAL PATHS AIDS PROJECT, Executive Director Kiyoshi Kuromiya, 2062 Lombard Street, Philadelphia, Pennsylvania 19146; telephone (212) 545-2212.
- DIRECT AIDS ALTERNATIVE INFORMATION

RESOURCES (DAAIR), Executive Director Fred Bingham, 31 East 30th Street, Suite 2A, New York, New York 10016; telephone (212) 725-6994; fax (212) 689-6471 (has a buyers club too).

- TOTAL HEALTH, joint Executive Directors Karen Masterson and Keith D. Vrhel, P.O. Box 60008, San Diego, California 92166; telephone (619) 296-6471.
- THE HIPPOCRATIC MEDICAL FOUNDATION, Executive Director Samuel Murdock, 10529 Sheldon Road, Elk Grove, California 95624.
- *AIDS Treatment News,* Editor John S. James, P.O. Box 411256, San Francisco, California 94141; telephone (415) 255-0588 or (415) 861-2432.
- GAY MEN'S HEALTH CRISIS, *Treatment Issues,* 129 West 20th Street, New York, New York 10011; fax (212) 337-3656.
- PROJECT INFORM, *PI Perspective,* 1965 Market Street, Suite 220, San Francisco, California 94103; telephone (415) 558-9051.
- SAN FRANCISCO AIDS FOUNDATION, *Bulletin of Experimental Treatments for AIDS (BETA),* P.O. Box 426182, San Francisco, California 94142; telephone (800) 327-9893.
- TEST POSITIVE AWARE NETWORK, Inc., *Positively Aware,* 1340 Irving Park, P.O. Box 259, Chicago, Illinois 60613.
- SEATTLE TREATMENT EDUCATION PROJECT, *Step Pespective,* 127 Broadway East, Suite 200, Seattle, Washington 98102; telephone (800) 869-7837.
- COMMUNITY AIDS TREATMENT INFORMATION EXCHANGE, *Treatment Update,* Suite 324, 517 College Street, Toronto, Ontario Canada M6G 4A2; telephone (416) 944-1916.
- NEWSLINE COALITION, Inc., Editor Bree Scott-Hartland, *PWA Newsline,* 31 West 26th Street, New York, New York 10010; telephone (212) 532-0290.
- PWA HEALTH GROUP, *Notes from the Under-*

ground, 150 West 26th Street, Suite 201, New York, New York 10001; telephone (212) 255-0520.

- ACT-UP/NEW YORK, *Treatment and Data Digest,* 135 West 29th Street, New York, New York 10001; telephone (212) 564-AIDS.
- AIDS PROJECT LOS ANGELES, Editor Stephan Korsia, *I Heard It Through the Grapevine,* 6721 Romaine Street, Los Angeles, California 90038.
- WORLD, Executive Director Rebecca Denison, P.O. Box 11535, Oakland, California 94611; telephone (510) 658-6930.
- THE POSITIVE WOMAN, P.O. Box 34372, Washington, District of Columbia 20043; telephone (202) 898-0372.
- SEARCH ALLIANCE, *Searchlight,* 7461 Beverly Boulevard, Suite 304, Los Angeles, California 90036; telephone (213) 930-8820; fax (213) 934-3919.
- BEING ALIVE, 3626 Sunset Boulevard, Los Angeles, California 90026; telephone (213) 667-3262.
- DALLAS GAY ALLIANCE, *AIDS Update,* P.O. Box 190712, Dallas, Texas 75219.
- BODY POSITIVE, Inc., *Body Positive,* 2095 Broadway, Suite 306, New York, New York 10023.
- BODY POSITIVE RESOURCE CENTER, *Up Front Drug Information,* 5701 Biscayne Boulevard, Suite 602, Miami, Florida 33137.

References

Introduction

1. Walker, M. "Olive leaf extract: The new oral treatment to counteract most types of pathological organisms." *Explore!* 7(4):31–37, Sept. 1996.

2. Dever, L. A., and Dermody, T. S. "Mechanisms of bacterial resistance to antibiotics." *Archives of Internal Medicine* 151:886–895, 1991.

3. Jacoby, G. A., and Archer, G. L. "New mechanisms of bacterial resistance to antimicrobial agents." *New England Journal of Medicine* 324:601–612, 1991.

4. Pooley, R. J., and Peterson, L. R. "Mechanisms of microbial susceptibility and resistance to antimicrobial agents." In *The Biologic and Clinical Basis of Infectious Diseases,* 5th edition. Editors S. T. Shulman, J. P. Phair, L. R. Peterson, and J. R. Warren (Philadelphia: W. B. Saunders Company, 1997), p. 550.

5. Sachs, J. S. "The drug resisters: Deadly new bacteria are shrugging off antibiotics." *Longevity,* April 1993, pp. 53–55.

6. Walker, M. "Antimicrobial attributes of olive leaf extract." *Townsend Letter for Doctors & Patients.* #156, July 1996, pp. 80–85.

Chapter 1

1. Stoffman, P.*The Family Guide to Preventing and Treating 100 Infectious Illnesses* (New York: John Wiley& Sons, Inc., 1995), p. 1.

2. Shulman, S. T. "Introduction to infectious diseases." In *The Biologic and Clinical Basis of Infectious Diseases,* 5th edition. Editors S. T. Shulman, J. P. Phair, L. R. Peterson, and J. R. Warren (Philadelphia: W. B. Saunders Company, 1997), p. 1.

3. Herceg, R. J., and Peterson, L. R. "Normal flora in health and disease." In *The Biologic and Clinical Basis of Infectious Diseases,* 5th edition. Editors S. T. Shulman, J. P. Phair, L. R. Peterson, and J. R. Warren (Philadelphia: W. B. Saunders Company, 1997), p. 13.

4. *Diseases,* 2nd edition (Springhouse, PA: Springhouse Corporation, 1997), p. 95.

5. *Professional Guide to Diseases,* 5th edition (Springhouse, PA: Springhouse Corporation, 1995), p. 145.

6. Ibid., p. 144.

7. Diseases, op. cit., p. 95.

8. Trowbridge, J. P., and Walker, M. *The Yeast Syndrome* (New York: Bantam Books, 1986), p. 39.

9. Emond, R. T. D.; Rowland, H. A. K.; Welsby, P. D. *Color Atlas of Infectious Diseases,* 3rd edition (London: Times Mirror International Publishers, Ltd., 1995), p. 7.

10. Brant, M.; Wingert, P.; Hager, M. "The end of antibiotics." *Newsweek,* March 28, 1994, pp. 47–51.

11. Stoffman, op. cit., p. 8.

12. Gittleman, A. L. *Guess What Came to Dinner: Parasites and Your Health* (Garden City Park, NY: Avery Publishing Group, Inc., 1993), p. 21.

13. Dubos, R. J. "The evolution and the ecology of microbial diseases. In *Bacterial and Mycotic Infections of Man* (3rd edition), editor René J. Dubos, (Philadelphia: J. B. Lippincott Co., 1958), pp. 14–27.

Chapter 2

1. Tranter, H. S.; Tassou, S. C.; Nychas, G. J. "The effect of ~~live~~ phenolic compound, oleuropein, on growth and entero- ~~production~~ by *Staphylococcus aureus. Journal of Applied* ~~7~~4:253–259, 1993.

2. Pasquale, A. D.; Monforte, M. T.; Calabro, M. L. "HPLC analysis of oleuropein and some flavonoids in leaf and bud of *Olea Europaea L. II Farmaco* 46(6):803–815, 1991.

3. Rosenblum, M. *Olives: The Life and Lore of a Noble Fruit* (New York: Farrar, Straus & Giroux, 1996), p. 55.

4. Renis, H. E. "In vitro antiviral activity of calcium elenolate." *Antimicrobial Agents and Chemotherapy* pp. 167–168, 1970.

5. Elliot, G. A.; Buthala, D. A.; DeYoung, E. N. "Preliminary safety studies with calcium elenolate, an antiviral agent." *Antimicrobial Agents and Chemotherapy* 173–176, 1969.

6. Trowbridge, J. P., and Walker, M. *The Yeast Syndrome* (New York: Bantam Books, 1986), pp. 132–133.

7. Baker, S. M. *Notes on the Yeast Problem* (New Haven: Gessell Institute of Human Development, 1985), p. 8.

8. Privitera, J. R. *Olive Leaf Extract: A New/Old Healing Bonanza for Manknd* (Covina, CA: NutriScreen, Inc., 1996).

9. Barilla, J. *Olive Oil Miracle: How the Mediterranean Marvel Helps Protect Against Arthritis, Heart Disease and Breast Cancer* (New Canaan, CT: Keats Publishing, Inc., 1996), pp. 43–44.

10. Ibid., pp. 36–38.

11. Simopoulos, A. P. "The Mediterranean food guide. Greek column rather than an Egyptian pyramid." *Nutrition Today* 30(2):54–61, 1995.

Chapter 3

1. Pallas, E. *Recueil de Memoires de Medecine, de Chirurgie, et de Pharmacie Militaires,* vol. xxiii (1827), p. 152.

2. Pallas, E. *Journal Universel des Sciences Medicales,* tome XIX, 1828, p. 257.

3. Pallas, E. *Recueil de Memoires de Medecine, de Chirurgie, et de Pharmacie Militaires,* vol. xxvi (1829), p. 159.

4. Petkov, V., and Manolov, P. "Pharmacological analysis of the iridoid oleuropein." *Arzneim.-Forsch. (Drug Research)* 22(9):1476–1486, Nov. 9, 1972.

5. Fleming, H. P.; Walter, W. M.; Etchells, J. L. "Antimicrobial properties of oleuropein and products of its hydrolysis from green olives." *Microbiology* 26(5):777–782, Nov. 1973.

6. Tassou, C. C.; Nychas, G. J. E.; Board, R. G. "Effect of phenolic compounds and oleuropein on the germination of *Bacillus cereus* T spores. *Biotechnology Applied Biochemistry* 13:231–237, 1991.

7. Elliott, G. A.; Buthala, D. A.; DeYoung, E. N. "Preliminary safety studies with calcium elenolate, an antiviral agent." *Antimicrobial Agents and Chemotherapy,* 1970, pp. 173–176.

8. Ibid., p. 176.

9. Tranter, H. S.; Tassou, S. C.; Nychas, G. J. "The effect of the olive phenolic compound, oleuropein, on growth and enterotoxin B production by *Staphylococcus aureus.*" *Journal of Applied Bacteriology* 74:253–259, 1993.

10. Vaugh, R. H., *in Industrial Fermentations,* Editors L. A. Underkofler and R. J. Hickey, Vol. 2 (New York: Chemical Publishing, 1954).

11. Noskin, G. A. "Nosocomial infections." In *The Biologic and Clinical Basis of Infectious Diseases,* 5th edition. Editors S. T. Shulman, J. P. Phair, L. R. Peterson, and J. R. Warren. (Philadelphia: W. B. Saunders Company, 1997), pp. 382–395.

12. Ibid., pp. 386–388.

13. Bourquelot, E., and Vintilesco, J. "Sur l'oleuropeinnouveau principle de nature glucosidique retire de l'olivier (*Olea europea* L.)." *Comptes Rendus Hebdomadaires des Seances de L'Academie des Sciences.* Paris, 147:533, 1908.

14. Juven, B.; Henis, Y.; Jacoby, B. "Studies on the mechanism of the antimicrobial action of oleuropein." *Journal of Applied Bacteriology* 35:559–567, 1972.

15. Harborne, J. B. "Phenolic glucosides and the natural distribution." In *Biochemistry of Phenolic Compounds,* editor J. B. Harborne, (London: Academic Press, 1964).

16. Fleming, Walter, Etchells, op. cit.

17. Gourama, H., and Bullerman, L. B. "Effects of oleuropein on growth and aflatoxin production by *Aspergillus parasiticus.*" Dept. Food Science & Technology, University of Nebraska, Lincoln, NE 68583–0919, 1987.

18. Tassou, C. C., and Nychas, G. J. E. "Inhibition of *Staphylococcus aureus* by olive phenolics in broth and in a model food system." *Journal of Food Protection* 57(2):120–124, Feb. 1994.

19. Tranter, H. S.; Tassou, S. C.; Nychas, G. J. "The effect of the olive phenolic compound, oleuropein, on growth and enterotoxin B production by *Staphylococcus aureus.*" *Journal of Applied Bacteriology* 74:253–259, 1993.

20. Nychas, G. J. E.; Tassou, S. C.; Board, R. G. *Letters in Applied Microbiology* 10:217–220, 1990.

21. Federici, F., and Bongi, G. "Improved method for isolation of bacterial inhibitors from oleuropein hydrolysis." *Applied and Environmental Microbiology.* 46(3):509–510, 1983.

22. Fleming, Walter, Etchells, op. cit.

Halstead, B. W. *The Scientific Basis of EDTA Chelation* Therapy. (Colton, CA: Golden Quill Publishers, Inc., 1979), p. 75.

Hanbury, D. "On the febrifuge properties of the olive *(Olea europaea,* L)" *Journal Universel des Sciences Medicales,* tome xix, p. 257.

Konlee, M. "The olive leaf." *Positive Health News,* No. 11, Spring 1996 (Keep Hope Alive, P.O. Box 27041, West Allis, WI 53227).

Pasquale, A. D.; Monforte, M. T.; Calabro, M. L. "HPLC analysis of oleuropein and some flavonoids in leaf and bud of *Olea europaea* L. *Il Pharmaco* 46(6):803–816, 1991.

Petkov and Manolov, op. cit.

Renis, H. E. "In vitro antiviral activity of calcium elenolate." *Antimicrobial Agents and Chemotherapy,* pp. 167–168, 1970.

Tassou, C. C.; Nychas, G. J. E.; Board, R. G. "Effect of phenolic compounds and oleuropein on the germination of *Bacillus cereus* T spores. *Biotechnology Applied Biochemistry* 13:231–237, 1991.

Tranter, Tassou, Nychas, op. cit.

Tutour, B. L., and Guedon, D. "Antioxidative activities of *Olea europaea* leaves and related phenolic compounds." *Phytochemistry* 31(4):1173–1178, 1992.

Vaugh, R. H., in *Industrial Fermentations,* editors L. A. Underkofler and R. J. Hickey, Vol. 2 (New York: Chemical Publishing, 1954).

23. Dring, G. J., and Gould, G. W. *Journal of General Microbiology* 65:101–104, 1971.

Elliott, G. A.; Buthala, D. A.; DeYoung, E. N. "Preliminary safety studies with calcium elenolate, an antiviral agent." *Antimicrobial Agents and Chemotherapy,* 8:173–199, 1975.

Fleming, H. P., and Etchells, J. L. *Applied Microbiology* 15:1178–1184, 1967.

Fleming, H. P.; Walter, W. M.; Etchells, J. L. *Applied Microbiology* 18:856–860, 1969.

Gould, G. W.; Hitchins, A. D.; King, W. L. *Journal of General Microbiology* 44:293–302, 1966.

Heinze, J. E.; Hale, A. H.; Carl, P. L. "Specificity of the antiviral agent calcium elenolate.'' *Antimicrobial Agents and Chemotherapy* 8(4):421–425.

Juven, R. & Henis, Y. *Journal of Applied Bacteriology* 33:721–732, 1970.

Moreno, E.; Perez, J.; Ramos-Cormezana, A.; Martinez, J. *Microbios* 51:169–174, 1974.

Nychas, Tassou, Board, op. cit.

Paredes, M. J.; Moreno, E.; Ramos-Cormenzana, A.; Martinez, J. *Chemosphere* 16:1557–1564, 1987.

Paredes, M. J.; Monteolina-Sanchez, M.; Moreno, E.; Perez, J.; Ramos-Cormenzana, A.; Martinez, J. *Chemosphere* 15:659–664, 1986.

Paster, N.; Juven, B. J.; Harshemesh, H. *Journal of Applied Bacteriology* 64:293–297, 1988.

Renis, H. E. ''In vitro antiviral activity of calcium elenolate.'' *Antimicrobial Agents and Chemotherapy*, pp. 167–172, 1969.

Rodriguez, M. M.; Perez, J.; Romps-Cormenzana, A.; Martinez, J. *Journal of Applied Bacteriology* 64:219–225, 1988.

Ruiz-Barba, J. L.; Rios-Sanchez, R. M.; Fedriani-Iriso, C.; Olias, J. M.; Rios, J. L.; Jimenez-Diaz, R. *Syst. Appl. Microbiol.* 13:199–205, 1990.

Soret, M. G. ''Antiviral activity of calcium elenolate on parainfluenza infection of hamsters.'' *Antimicrobial Agents and Chemotherapy*, pp. 160–166, 1969.

Vazqeuz-Roncero, A.; Maestro Duran, M.; Graciani, Constante, E. *Grasas Aceites (Seville)* 25:341–345, 1974.

Chapter 4

1. Rosenblum, M. *Olives: The Life and Lore of a Noble Fruit* (New York: Farrar, Straus & Giroux, 1996), pp. 195–196.

2. Ibid., p. 196.

3. Asaka, Y.; Kamikawa, Tk.; Kubota, T.; Sakamoto, H. ''Structures of seco-iridoids from *Ligstrum obtusifolium.*'' *Chemical Letters* 00:141–144, 1972.

4. Kubo, I.; Matsumoto, A.; Takase, I. ''A multichemical defense mechanism of bitter olive *Olea europaea* (Oleaceae): Is oleuropein a phytoalexin precursor?'' *Journal of Chemical Ecology* 11(2):251–263, 1985.

5. De Whalley, C. V.; Rankin, S. M.; Hoult, J. R. S.; Jessup, W.; Leake, D. S. *Biochem Pharmacology* 39:1743–1750, 1990.

Elliot, G. A.; Buthala, D. A.; DeYoung, E. N. "Preliminary safety studies with calcium elenolate, an antiviral agent." *Antimicrobial Agents and Chemotherapy* 173–176, 1969.

Fleming, H. P., and Etchells, J. L. "Occurrence of inhibitor of lactic acid bacteria in green olives." *Applied Microbiology* 14:1178–1184, 1967.

Fleming, H. P.; Walter, W. M.; Etchells, J. L. *Applied Microbiology* 18:859–860, 1969.

Hertog, M. G. L.; Feskens, E. J. M.; Hollman, P. C. H.; Katan, M. B.; Kromhout, D. *Lancet* 342:1007–1011, 1993.

Inven, B., and Henis, Y. *Journal of Applied Bacteriology* 33:721–732, 1970.

Kunhau, J. *World Revue of Nutrition and Diet* 24:117–191, 1976.

Moreno, E.; Perez, J.; Ramos-Cormezana, A.; Martinez, J. *Microbios* 51:169–174, 1987.

Mortimer, P. R., and McCann, G. "Food poisoning episodes associated with *Bacillus cereus* in fried rice." *Lancet* 1:1043–1045, 1974.

Nychas, G. J. E.; Tassou, S. C.; Board, R. G. *Letters in Applied Microbiology* 10:217–220, 1990.

Paredes, M. J.; Monteleolina-Sanchez, M.; Moreno, E.; Perez, J.; Ramos-Cormenzana, A.; Martinez, J. *Chemosphere* 15:659–664, 1986.

Paredes, M. J.; Moreno, E.; Ramos-Cormenzana, A.; Martinez, J. *Chemosphere* 16:1557–1564, 1987.

Parker, M. S., and Bradley, M. J. *Canadian Journal of Microbiology* 141:745–746, 1968.

Pasquale, A. D.; Monforte, M. T.; Calabro, M. L. "HPLC analysis of oleuropein and some flavonoids in leaf and bud of *Olea europaea L.*" *Il Farmaco* 46(6):803–815, 1991.

Paster, N.; Juven, B. J.; Harshemesh, H. *Journal of Applied Bacteriology* 64:293–297, 1988.

Renis, H. E. "In vitro antiviral activity of calcium elenolate." *Antimicrobial Agents and Chemotherapy* pp. 167–168, 1970.

Rodriguez, M. M.; Perez, J.; Romps-Cormenzana, A.; Martinez, J. *Journal of Applied Bacteriology* 64:219–225, 1988.

Rutz-Barba, J. L.; Rios-Sanchez, R. M.; Fedriant-Iriso, C.; Olias, J. M.; Rios, J. L.; Ji-Menez, Diaz, R. *System Applied Microbiology* 13:199–205, 1990.

Sierra, G. *Canadian Journal of Microbiol* 16:51–52, 1970.

Tassou, C. C.; Nychas, G. J. E.; Board, R. G. "Effect of phenolic compounds and oleuropein on the germination of *Bacillus cereus* T spores." *Biotechnology Applied Biochemistry* 13:231–237, 1991.

Tranter, H. S.; Tassou, S. C.; Nychas, G. J. "The effect of the olive phenolic compound, oleuropein, on growth and enterotoxin B production by *Staphylococcus aureus*. *Journal Applied Bacteriology* 74:253–259, 1993.

Vaughn, R. H., in *Industrial Fermentations,* Editors L. A. Underkotler, and R. J. Hickey, Vol. 2 (New York: Chemical Publishing, 1954).

Vazquez-Roncero, A.; Maestro Duran, M.; Graciani, C. E. *Grrasas Aceites.* 25:341–345, 1974.

Visioli, F., and Galli, C. "Oleuropein protects low density lipoprotein from oxidation." *Life Sciences* 55(24):1965–1971, 1994.

Visioli, F.; Vinceri, F. F.; Galli, C. *"Waste waters' from olive oil production are rich in natural antioxidants* (Basel: Virkhauser Verlag, 1995), p. 32–34.

Chapter 5

1. Petkov, V., and Manolov, P. "Pharmacological studies on substances of plant origin with coronary dilatating and antiarrhythmic action." *Comparative Medicine East and West* VI(2):123–130, 1978.

2. Ibid., p. 130.

3. Zarzuelo, A.; Duarte, J.; Jimenez, J.; Gonzales, M.; Utrilla, M. P. "Vasodilator effect of olive leaf." *Planta Medicine* 57:417–419, 1991.

4. Petkov, V., and Manolov, P. "Pharmacological analysis of the iridoid oleuropein." *Arzneim.-Forsch. (Drug Research)* 22:1476–141486, Nov. 9, 1972.

5. Ibid., pp. 1478–1479.

6. Petkov, V. "Plants with hypotensive, antiatheromatous and coronarodilatating action." *American Journal of Chinese Medicine* VII(3):197–236, 1979.

7. Samuelsonn, G. "The blood pressure lowering factor in leaves of *Olea europaea.*" *Farmacevitisk Revy* 15:229–239, 1951.

8. Panizzi, L., et al. "The constitution of oleuropein, a bitter glucoside of the olive with hypotensive action." *Gass. Chim. Ital.* 90:1449–1485, 1960.

9. *The Merck Manual,* 16th edition (Rahway, NJ: Merck & Co., 1992), p. 475.

10. Walker, M. "Antimicrobial attributes of olive leaf extract." *Townsend Letter for Doctors & Patients,* #156, July 1996, pp. 80–85.

11. Walker, M. "Olive leaf extract: The new oral treatment to counteract most types of pathological organisms." *Explore! for the Professional* 7(4):31–37, Nov. 1996.

12. Visioli, F., and Galli, C. "Oleuropein protects low density lipoprotein from oxidation." *Life Sciences* 55(24):1865–1971, 1994.

13. Ruiz-Gutierrez, V.; Muriana, F. J. G.; Maestro, R.; Graciani, E. "Oleuropein on lipid and fatty acid composition of rat heart." *Nutrition Research* 15(1):37–51, 1995.

14. Kunhau, J. *World Revue of Nutrition and Diet* 24:117–191, 1976.

15. De Whalley, C. V.; Rankin, S. M.; Hoult, J. R. S.; Jessup, W.; Leake, D.S. *Biochemistry and Pharmacology* 39:1743–1750, 1990.

16. Hertog, M. G. L.; Feskens, E. J. M.; Hollman, P. C. H.; Katan, M. B.; Kromhout, D. *Lancet* 342:1007–1011, 1993.

17. Visioli, F.; Vinceri, F. F.; Galli, C. *"Waste waters" from olive oil production are rich in natural antioxidants* (Basel: Virkhauser Verlag, 1995), pp. 32–34.

18. Tutour, B. L., and Guedon, D. "Antoxidative activities of *Olea europaea* leaves and related phenolic compounds." *Phytochemistry* 31(4):1173–1178, 1992.

19. Privitera, J. R. *Olive Leaf Extract—A New/Old Healing Bonanza for Mankind* (Covina, California: James R. Privitera, 1996), p. 33.

Chapter 6

1. *The Merck Manual,* 16th edition (Rahway, NJ: Merck & Co., Inc., 1992), pp. 270–271.

2. Weiner, M. A. *Maximum Immunity* (Bath, England: Gateway Books, 1986), pp. 145–149.

3. Emond, R. T. D.; Rowland, H. A. K.; Welsby, P. D. *Color Atlas of Infectious Diseases,* 3rd edition (London: Mosby-Wolfe, 1995), p. 204.

4. *Professional Guide to Diseases,* 5th edition (Springhouse, PA: Springhouse Corporation, 1995), p. 216.

5. Kennedy, R. P. *Herpes: How to Live with It; How to Treat It; How Not to Treat It.* (Santa Barbara, CA: American Medical Publishing Co., 1983), pp. 6–12.

6. Konlee, M. *How to Reverse Immune Dysfunction,* 5th edition. (West Allis, WI: Keep Hope Alive, 1996), p. 11.

7. Tedder, R.; Briggs, M.; Cameron, C. H.; Honess, R.; Robertson, D.; Whittle, H. "A novel lymphotropic herpesvirus." *Lancet* 2:390–392, 1987.

8. Fox, J. D.; Briggs, M.; Ward, P. A., et al. "Human herpesvirus 6 in salivary glands." *Lancet* 336:590–594, 1990.

Harnett, G. E.; Farr, T. J.; Pietroboni, G. R., et al. "Frequent shedding of HHV-6 in saliva. *J. Med. Virol.* 30:128–130, 1990.

9. Levine, Arnold J. *Viruses* (New York: Scientific American Library, 1992), pp. 84–85.

10. Tanaka, K.; Kondo, T.; Torigoe, S.; Okada, S.; Mukai, T.; Yamanishi, K. "Human herpesvirus 7: Another casual agent for roseola (exanthem subitum)." *Journal of Pediatrics* 125(1):1–5, July 1994.

11. Renis, H. E. "In vitro antiviral activity of calcium elenolate." *Antimicrobial Agents and Chemotherapy,* 1970, pp. 167–171.

12. Kaij-a-Kamb, M.; Amoros, M.; Girre, L. "Search for new antiviral agents of plant origin." *Pharma-Acta-Helv,* 67(5–6):130–147, 1992.

Chapter 7

1. Holms, Gary, P.; Kaplan, Jonathan E.; Gantz, Nelson M.; Komaroff, Anthony L.; Schonberger, Lawrence B.; Straus, Stephen E.; Jones, James F.; Dubois, Richard E.; Cunningham-Rundles, Charlotte; Pahwa, Savita; Tosato, Giovanna; Zegans, Leonard S.; Purtilo, David T.; Brown, Nathaniel; Schooley, Robert T.; and Brus, Irena. "Chronic fatigue syndrome: A working case definition." *Annals of Internal Medicine* 108:387–389, 1988.

Jaret, Peter. "Chronic fatigue syndrome: An update." *Glamour,* Nov. 1992.

Petersdorf, R. G.; Adams, R. D.; Braunwald, E.; et al. *Har-*

rison's Principles of Internal Medicine 10th Edition (New York: McGraw-Hill, 1983).

2. Jones, J. F.; Ray, G.; Minnich, L. L.; et al. "Evidence for active Epstein-Barr virus infection in patients with persistent unexplained illness: Elevated anti-early antigen antibodies." *Annals of Internal Medicine* 102:1–7, 1985.

Strauch, B.; Andrews, L.; Miller, G.; et al. "Oropharyngeal excretion of Epstein-Barr virus by renal transplant recipients and other patients treated with immunosuppression drugs." *Lancet* i:234, 1974.

Straus, S. E.; Tosato, F.; Armstrong, G.; et al. "Persisting illness and fatigue in adults with evidence of Epstein-Barr virus infection." *Annals of Internal Medicine* 102:7–16, 1985.

3. Dubois, R. E.; Seely, J. R.; Brus, I.; et al. "Chronic mononucleosis syndrome." *South. Med. J.* 77:1376–1382, 1984.

Jones, J. F. "Chronic Epstein-Barr virus infection in children." *Pediatric Infectious Disease* 5:503–504, 1986.

Sixbey, J. W.; Nedrud, J. G.; Raab-Traub, N.; Hanes, R. A.; Pagano, J. S. "Epstein-Barr virus replication in oropharyngeal epithelial cells." *New England Journal of Medicine* 310:1225–1230, 1984.

Tobi, M.; Morag, A.; Ravid, Z.; et al. "Prolonged atypical illness associated with serological evidence of persistent Epstein-Barr virus infection." *Lancet* i:61–64, 1982.

4. Andiman, W. A. "The Epstein-Barr virus infections in childhood." *Journal of Pediatrics* 95:171, 1979.

Rapp, C. E., and J. F. Hewetson. "Infectious mononucleosis and the Epstein-Barr virus." *American Journal of Disease Children* 132:78, 1978.

5. Henle, W.; Henle, G.; Lennette, E. T. "The Epstein-Barr virus." *Scientific American* 241:48, 1979.

6. Miller, G.; Niederman, J. D.; Andrews, L. "Prolonged oropharyngeal excretion of Epstein-Barr virus after infectious mononucleosis." *New England Journal of Medicine* 288:229, 1973.

Rocchi, G.; DeFelici, A.; Ragona, G.; et al. "Quantitative evaluation of Epstein-Barr virus-infected mononuclear peripheral blood leukocytes in infectious mononucleosis." *New England Journal of Medicine* 296:132, 1977.

7. Donovan, Patrick M. "Chronic mononucleosis-like syndrome: Primary EBV infection or indicator of immune system dysfunction?" In Pizzorno and Murray, *Chronic Mononucleosis*, Nov. 16, 1987, p. 1.

8. Henig, Robin Marantz. *A Dancing Matrix: Voyages Along the Viral Frontier*. (New York: Alfred A. Knopf, 1993), pp. 58–61.

9. Gallo, Robert. *Virus Hunting: AIDS, Cancer, and the Human Retrovirus: A Story of Scientific Discovery*. (New York: Basic Books, 1991), p. 96.

10. Winslow, Ron. "Virus may have role in causing chronic fatigue." *The Wall Street Journal*, September 16, 1991.

11. Cowley, Geoffrey and Mary Hager. "A clue to chronic fatigue." *Newsweek*, Lifestyle-Medicine Section, 1991.

12. Renis, H. E. "In vitro antiviral activity of calcium elenolate." *Antimicrobial Agents and Chemotherapy* 167–172, 1970.

Chapter 8

1. Brink, W. D. "Reexamining AIDS/potential non-toxic protocols." *Townsend Letter for Doctors & Patients*, pp. 50–53, Dec. 1996.

2. Sherman, W. "Selling vials of hope." *Longevity*, March 1992, pp. 61–69.

3. Arno, P. S., and Feiden, K.L. *Against the Odds: The Story of AIDS Drug Development, Politics and Profit* (New York: HarperCollins, 1992).

4. "Scientist reports that HIV in the presence of HHV-6A replicates 10 to 15 times faster." *Positive Health News*, Report No. 10, Winter 1995, p. 11.

5. Duesberg, P. H. "AIDS epidemiology: Inconsistencies with human immunodeficiency virus and with infectious disease." *Proceedings of the National Academy of Science* 88:1575–1579, 1991.

Duesberg, P. H. "Human immunodeficiency virus and acquired immunodeficiency syndrome: Correlation but not causation." *Proceedings of the National Academy of Science* 86:755–764, 1989.

6. The American Academy for the Advancement of Science conference, June 22, 1995, San Francisco State University.

7. Benjamini, E., and Leskowitz, S. *Immunology: A Short Course* (New York: John Wiley & Sons, Inc., 1991), p. 154.

8. Konlee, M. "Protease inhibitors—Back to 'Eden.'" *Positive Health News* 11:2, Spring 1996.

9. Ibid., p. 14.

10. Konlee, M. *How to Reverse Immune Dysfunction* (West Allis, WI: Keep Hope Alive, 1996).

Chapter 9

1. Beyerman, H. C.; van Dijck, L. A.; Levisalles, J.; Melera, A.; Veer, W.L.C. *Bulletin of Science and Chemistry. France.* 10:1812 1961.

2. Soret, op. cit.
Hirschman, S. Z. *Science* 173:441 1971.

3. Hirschman, op. cit.
Panizzi, L.; Scarpati, M. L.; Oriente, G. *Gazz. Chim. Ital.* 90:1449 1960.

4. Hirschman, S. Z. "Inactivation of DNA polymerases of murine leukaemia viruses by calcium elenolate." *Nature New Biology* 238:277–279 August 30, 1972.
Renis, H. E. "Influenza virus infection of hamsters. A model for evaluating antiviral drugs." *Antimicrobial Agents and Chemotherapy* 167 (American Society for Microbiology 1969).

5. Mills, J. "What's new about the common cold? Results of surprising studies." *Modern Medicine* November 1981.
Soret, M. G. "Antiviral activity of calcium elenolate on parainfluenza infection of hamsters." *Antimicrobial Agents and Chemotherapy* 160 (American Society for Microbiology 1969).

6. Renis, H. E. "Inactivation of myxoviruses by calcium elenolate." *Antimicrobial Agents and Chemotherapy* pp. 194–199 August 1975.
Renis, H. E. *"In vitro* antiviral activity of calcium elenolate." *Antimicrobial Agents and Chemotherapy* pp. 167–172 1969.

7. Stoffman, P. *The Family Guide to Preventing & Treating 100 Infectious Illnesses.* (New York: John Wiley & Sons Inc. 1995) p. 153.

8. Renis, H. E. "Influenza virus infection of hamsters. A model for evaluating antiviral drugs." *Archives of Virology* 54:85–93 1977.

9. Katz, B. Z. and Thomson, R. B. "Viral infections of the lower respiratory tract." In *The Biologic and Clinical Basis of Infectious Diseases* 5th edition. Editors S. T. Shulman J. P. Phair L. R. Peterson J. R. Warren (Philadelphia: W. B. Saunders Co. 1997) pp. 143–156.

10. Renis, op. cit. 1975.

11. Renis, op. cit. 1969.

12. Till, M. "Viral infections of the central nervous system." In *The Biologic and Clinical Basis of Infectious Diseases* 5th edition. Editors S. T. Shulman J. P. Phair L. R. Peterson J. R. Warren (Philadelphia: W. B. Saunders Co. 1997) pp. 327–343.

13. Stoffman op. cit., pp. 248–251.

Chapter 10

1. Mcarty, M. "The hemolytic streptococci." In *Bacterial and Mycotic Infections of Man,* 3rd edition, editor René J. Dubos (Philadelphia: J. B. Lippincott Company, 1958), p. 248.

2. Warren, J. R. "Bacteria-host interactions." In *The Biologic and Clinical Basis of Infectious Diseases,* 5th edition. Editors S. T. Shulman, J. P. Phair, L. R. Peterson, J. R. Warren (Philadelphia: W. B. Saunders Co., 1997), pp. 29–30.

3. Fleming, H. P., and Etchells, J. L. "Occurrence of inhibitor of lactic acid bacteria in green olives." *Applied Microbiology* 14:1178–1184, 1967.

Vaughn, R. H. in *Industrial Fermentations.* Editors L. A. Underkotler, and R. J. Hickey, Vol. 2 (New York: Chemical Publishing, 1954).

4. Fleming, H. P.; Walter, W. M.; Etchells, J. L. *Applied Microbiology* 18:859–860, 1969.

Rutz-Barba, J. L.; Rios-Sanchez, R. M.; Fedriant-Iriso, C.; Olias, J. M.; Rios, J. L.; Ji-Menez, Diaz, R. *Syst. Applied Microbiology* 13:199–205, 1990.

5. Vazqeuz-Roncero, A.; Maestro Duran, M.; Graciani, C. E. *Grasas Aceites* 25:341–345, 1974.

6. Moreno, E.; Perez, J.; Ramos-Cormezana, A.; Martinez, J. *Microbios* 51:169–174, 1987.

7. Paredes, M. J.; Monteleolina-Sanchez, M.; Moreno, E.; Perez, J.; Ramos-Cormenzana, A.; Martinez, J. *Chemosphere* 15:659–664, 1986.

Paredes, M. J.; Moreno, E.; Ramos-Cormenzana, A.; Martinez, J. *Chemosphere* 16:1557–1564, 1987.

8. Rodriguez, M. M.; Perez, J.; Romps-Cormenzana, A.; Martinez, J. *Journal of Applied Bacteriology* 64:219–225.

9. Inven, B., and Henis, Y. *Journal of Applied Bacteriology* 33:721–732, 1970.

Paster, N.; Juven, B. J.; Harshemesh, H. *Journal of Applied Bacteriology* 64:293–297, 1988.

10. Nychas, G. J. E.; Tassou, S. C.; Board, R. G. *Letters in Applied Microbiology* 10:217–220, 1990.

11. Elliott, G. A.; Buthala, D. A.; DeYoung, E. N. "Preliminary safety studies with calcium elenolate, an antiviral agent." *Antimicrobial Agents and Chemotherapy,* American Society for Microbiology, 1970.

12. Walker, M. "Dr. William Donald Kelley charges contamination of pancreatic enzymes." *Townsend Letter for Doctors* 65:535–551, Dec. 1988.

13. Mortimer, P. R., and McCann, G. "Food poisoning episodes associated with *Bacillus cereus* in fried rice." *Lancet* 1:1043–1045, 1974.

14. Walker, op. cit., pp. 547–548.

15. Tassou, C. C.; Nychas, G. J. E.; Board, R. G. "Effect of phenolic compounds and oleuropein on the germination of *Bacillus cereus* T spores." *Biotechnology Applied Biochemistry* 13:231–237, 1991.

16. Parker, M. S. and Bradley, M.J. *Canadian Journal of Microbiology* 141:745–746, 1968.

17. Sierra, G. *Canadian Journal of Microbiology* 16:51–52, 1970.

18. Bourquelot, E., and Vintilesco, J. *Canadian Royal Academy of Sciences* 147:533–535, 1908.

Creuss, W. V., and Alsberg, C. L. *Journal of the American Chemical Society* 56:2115–2117, 1934.

Fleming, H. P., et al. *Applied Microbiology* 26(5):773–782, 1973.

Kubo, I., et al. *Journal of Chemical Ecology* 11(2):251–263, 1985.

Panizzi, L., et al. *Gazz. Chim. Ital.* 90:1449–1485, 1960.

Petkov, V., and Manolov, P. *Drug Research* 22(9):1476–1486, 1972.

19. Gariboldi, P., et al. *Phytochemistry* 25(4):865–869, 1986.

Kelley, R. C., et al. *Journal of the American Chemical Society* 95(21):7155–7156, 1973.

Veer, W. L. C. U.S. Patent 3,033,877, 1962.

Veer, W. L. C., et al. *J. Rec. Trav. Chim. Pay Bas.* 76:839–840, 1957.

20. Fleming, op. cit., pp. 777–782.

Hirschman, S. Z. *Nature (New Biology)* 238:227–229, 1972.

Renis, H. E. *Antimicrobial Agents & Chemotherapy* 1970, pp. 167–172.

21. Elliot, G. A., et al. *Antimicrobial Agents & Chemotherapy,* 1970, pp. 173–176.

Soret, M.G. *Antimicrobial Agents & Chemotherapy,* 1970, pp. 160–166.

22. Creuss, W. V. *IV Congress International Tech. Chim. Ind. Agr.,* Brussels. 3:638–645, 1935.

Creuss and Alsberg, op. cit.

23. Gariboldi, P., op. cit.

Pizzalato, G., et al. *Tetrahedron* 44(11):3203–3208, 1988.

Chapter 11

1. Moss, E. S., and McQuown. *Atlas of Medical Mycology* (Baltimore: Williams & Wilkins Co., 1960).

2. Emond, R. T. D.; Rowland, H. A.; Welsby, P. D. *Color Atlas of Infectious Diseases,* 3rd edition (London: Mosby-Wolfe, 1995).

Hazen, E. L., and Reed, F. C. *Laboratory Identification of Pathogenic Fungi Simplified* (Springfield, IL: Charles C Thomas, 1960).

Jacobson, H. P. *Fungous Diseases: A Clinico-Mycological Text* (Springfield, IL: Charles C Thomas, 1932).

Moss & McQuown, op. cit., pp. 8–9.

3. Trowbridge, J. P., and Walker, M. *The Yeast Syndrome: How to Help Your Doctor Identify and Treat the Real Cause of Your Yeast-Related Illness* (New York: Bantam Books, 1986), pp. 72–77.

4. Trowbridge, J. P., and Walker, M. *Yeast-Related Illnesses* (Byram, NY: Devin-Adair, 1985).

5. Trowbridge & Walker, op cit.

6. Yutsis, P., and Walker, M. *The Downhill Syndrome: If Nothing's Wrong, Why Do I Feel So Bad? How to Overcome Generalized Tiredness, Disabling Fatigue or Outright Exhaustion and Restore High-Level Wellness to Your Body & Mind.* (Garden City Park, NY: Avery Publishing Group, Inc., 1997), pp. 83–84.

Chapter 12

1. Yutsis, P. I., and Walker, M. *The Downhill Syndrome* (Garden City Park, NY: Avery Publishing Group, Inc., 1997).
2. Gittleman, A. L. *Guess What Came to Dinner: Parasites and Your Health* (Garden City Park, NY: Avery Publishing Group, Inc., 1993).
3. Kristoff, N. D. "Malaria makes a comeback, and is more deadly than ever." *The New York Times,* Vol. CXLLVI, No. 50,666, January 8, 1997, p. A1.

Chapter 13

1. U. S. Congress, General Accounting Office, *Automated Medical Records: Leadership Needed to Expedite Standards Development* (Washington, DC: General Accounting Office, 1993).
2. Kubo, I., et al. "A multichemical defense mechanism of bitter olive *Olea europaea* (Oleaceae)—Is oleuropein a phytoalexin precursor?" *Journal of Chemistry & Ecology* 11(2):251–263, 1985.
3. Heinze, J. E., et al. "Specificity of the antiviral agent calcium elenolate." *Antimicrobial Agents in Chemotherapy* 8(4):421–425, 1975.

Juven, B., et al. "Studies on the mechanism of the antimicrobial action of oleuropein." *Journal of Applied Bacteriology* 35:559–567, 1972.
4. Panizzi, L., et al. "The constitution of oleuropein, a bitter glucoside of the olive with hypotensive action." *Gazz. Chim. Ital.* 1449–1485, 1960.

Samuelsson, G. "The blood pressure lowering factor in leaves of *Olea europaea.*" *Farmacevtisk Revy* 15:229–239.
5. Visoli, F., and Galli, C. "Oleuropein protects low density lipoprotein from oxidation." *Life Sciences* 55(24):1965–1971, 1994.
6. "Researchers find how disease-resistant plants recognize bacteria." Press release, Purdue News, December 20, 1996.
7. Fredrickson, W. R. "A study of the efficacy of the olive preparation *Tinctura Olea foliorum* in treatment of herpetic infection." *Townsend Letter for Doctors & Patients* 166:110–111, May 1997.
8. Stephenson, J. "Investigators seeking new ways to stem rising tide of resistant fungi." *Journal of the American Medical Association* 277(1):5–6, Jan. 1, 1997.

About the Author

MORTON WALKER, D.P.M. A doctor of podiatric medicine, Dr. Morton Walker now writes full-time as a professional freelance medical journalist. He has published sixty-nine books (including twelve 100,000-copy bestsellers) and nearly 1,900 consumer magazine, clinical journal, and newspaper articles. Each month, he writes columns for five medically oriented periodicals: two American holistic clinical journals, two consumer health magazines, and a trade journal of the health foods industry. His books are published in twenty-eight countries, and the number continues to grow.

Dr. Walker has been featured by, or appeared as a guest with, Regis Philbin and Kathie Lee Gifford, Oprah Winfrey, Mike Douglas, Merv Griffin, Sally Jessy Raphael, Jay Leno, and other television talk show hosts. Dr. Walker specializes in those health care sciences referred to as orthomolecular nutrition, holistic (biological) medicine, and alternative methods of healing.

The winner of twenty-three (23) medical journalism awards and medals, Dr. Walker was recognized with the 1992 *Humanitarian Award* from the American Cancer Control Society, which named him: "The world's leading medical journalist specializing in holistic medicine."

He received the 1981 *Orthomolecular Award* from the American Institute of Preventive Medicine, for his "outstanding achievement in orthomolecular education."

He was presented with the 1979 *Humanitarian Award* from the 1,100 physician-members of the American College for Advancement in Medicine "for informing the American public on alternative methods of healing."

He has received two prestigious Jesse H. Neal *Editorial Achievement Awards* from the American Business Press, Inc., for creating the best series of magazine articles published in any audited United States magazine in both 1975 and 1976.